Soft Tissue and Trigger Point Release

Hands-On Guides for Therapists

Second Edition

Jane Johnson, MSc

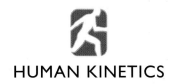

HUMAN KINETICS

Library of Congress Cataloging-in-Publication Data

Names: Johnson, Jane, 1965- author.
Title: Soft tissue and trigger point release / Jane Johnson.
Other titles: Soft tissue release
Description: Second edition. | Champaign : Human Kinetics, 2019. | Series:
  Hands-on guides for therapists | Preceded by Soft tissue release / Jane
  Johnson. 2009. | Includes bibliographical references. |
  Identifiers: LCCN 2018016640 (print) | LCCN 2018017346 (ebook) | ISBN
  9781492567639 (e-book) | ISBN 9781492567622 (print)
Subjects: | MESH: Massage--methods
Classification: LCC RM721 (ebook) | LCC RM721 (print) | NLM WB 537 | DDC
  615.8/22--dc23
LC record available at https://lccn.loc.gov/2018016640

ISBN: 978-1-4925-6762-2 (print)

The web addresses cited in this text were current as of May 2018, unless otherwise noted.

Senior Acquisitions Editor: Joshua J. Stone; **Developmental Editor:** Melissa J. Zavala; **Managing Editor:** Anne E. Mrozek; **Copyeditor:** Joanna Hatzopoulos Portman; **Senior Graphic Designer:** Joe Buck; **Cover Designer:** Keri Evans; **Cover Design Associate:** Susan Rothermel Allen; **Photograph (cover):** © Human Kinetics; **Photographs (interior):** © Human Kinetics; **Photo Production Coordinator:** Amy M. Rose; **Photo Production Manager:** Jason Allen; **Senior Art Manager:** Kelly Hendren; **Art Style Development:** Joanne Brummett; **Illustrations:** © Human Kinetics; **Printer:** Versa Press

Printed in the United States of America

10 9 8 7 6 5 4 3 2 1

The paper in this book is certified under a sustainable forestry program.

Human Kinetics

P.O. Box 5076
Champaign, IL 61825-5076
Website: www.HumanKinetics.com

In the United States, email info@hkusa.com or call 800-747-4457.
In Canada, email info@hkcanada.com.
In the United Kingdom/Europe, email hk@hkeurope.com.

For information about Human Kinetics' coverage in other areas of the world, please visit our website: **www.HumanKinetics.com**

E7319

The updated and revised edition of *Soft Tissue Release* is again dedicated to my son, Jake Johnson, who was 10 years old at the time the first edition was published. He has now reached the age of 19 and seems unscathed by having been brought up by a less than conventional mother. I am every day grateful to have him in my life.

Contents

4 Active-Assisted Soft Tissue Release   59

5 Active Soft Tissue Release   93

PART III Applying Soft Tissue Release

8   Soft Tissue Release for the Upper Limbs   199

PART IV   Soft Tissue Release Programmes

The Hands-On Guides for Therapists series was originally developed to provide the best clinical and educational resources for massage therapists, who were growing in number but for whom scant material existed to support the techniques they were learning and using. *Soft Tissue Release*, *Deep Tissue Massage* and *Sports Massage* were the first titles to be published for this growing market. They proved so popular that they were soon followed by *Therapeutic Stretching* and *Myofascial Release*. As professionals from other disciplines began to use and enjoy the material in this series, the range of titles was expanded to include *Postural Assessment* and *Postural Correction,* appealing particularly to students of physiotherapy, osteopathy and chiropractic, as well as to sports therapists, fitness instructors and teachers of yoga and Pilates.

The core focus of the Hands-On Guides for Therapists series remains the provision of specific tools of assessment and treatment that may be utilized by bodyworkers. Each book in the series contains simple explanations of a technique, often using a step-by-step approach, and full colour photographs throughout. With many years' experience, authors have provided tips containing handy advice to help therapists adjust their technique to help them become proficient. Client Talk boxes contain examples of how the techniques have been used with clients who have particular problems. At the end of each chapter are questions that enable readers to test their knowledge and skill, particularly helpful for those about to sit exams in the subject. Answers are provided at the back of the book.

Information in the Hands-On Guides for Therapists series has also proved useful for course tutors who have used these titles as textbooks to support courses in these subjects.

Postural Assessment and *Postural Correction* are each supported by an online CE course that, once completed, provides CE credits for a wide variety of governing bodies. Similar courses are being developed for other titles in the series.

Written for all therapists wishing to add to their existing soft tissue skills, the first edition of *Soft Tissue Release* was published in 2009. Designed to be used as a stand-alone text, with photographs supporting the step-by-step explanations, the first edition proved to be a valuable support text for therapists attending workshops in soft tissue release (STR) or studying on longer courses where STR formed one of the modules, such as sports massage therapy. Therapists who were already trained in the technique found it a helpful reference. Because this form of stretching may also be performed through clothing, fitness instructors, sport coaches, sport therapists, physiotherapists, osteopaths, chiropractors and other bodyworkers were also able to utilize this material.

Almost 10 years since publication of this hands-on guide, the new edition of *Soft Tissue Release* builds on the original text with the addition of text, photographs, illustrations and tables. One of the most significant additions is material describing how STR may be used to deactivate trigger points.

Introductory chapter 1 provides answers to common questions about use of the technique, such as How does the technique work? Who should have it? Where and when should it be applied? and What are the benefits of the technique? This chapter has two new sections, one describing the use of STR technique for deactivating trigger points and one about current research on the topic of stretching. The new section on trigger points describes what they are, why they should be treated, how to identify them and how to use STR to deactivate them. To clarify these points, eight photographs have been added to the step-by-step description of passive STR.

Chapter 2 is about preparing for STR, and it has new photographs illustrating additional handholds and methods of locking tissues. An illustration of the visual analogue scale (VAS) has been added, plus photographs of simple muscle length tests have been added to the section on measuring your effectiveness.

Chapters 3, 4 and 5 provide detailed information about how to apply different forms of STR: passive, active-assisted and active, respectively. Within each of these chapters three new sections have been added: the direction of locks, how to take up slack in the skin and the direction of pressure. Arrows have been added to photographs in each of these chapters to show in which direction pressure needs to be applied in order to take up slack in tissues as a lock is applied. Each chapter now has a section about how to use that form of STR to deactivate trigger points.

In addition, each chapter has an overview table with thumbnail photographs showing all of the techniques described in that chapter. The reader may use it as a checklist when learning to use STR. Finally, each chapter has a new section with ideas for how to become proficient in the use of that particular form of STR.

Chapter 3 has new photographs and illustrations as well as a new section describing how to apply passive STR to shoulder adductors.

Chapter 4 has new photographs and illustrations. In addition, a new table shows which muscles are usually treated in a neutral position and which are usually shortened. A new section describes how to incorporate active-assisted STR into an oil massage, and a new form of this technique is introduced—gliding STR. New sections have been added describing active-assisted STR to the iliotibial band (ITB), infraspinatus, biceps brachii and triceps.

Chapter 5 has new photos and illustrations plus new sections describing how to apply active STR to gluteals, trapezius, scalenes, rhomboid and pectoral muscles.

Part III contains three chapters, each focusing on the application of STR to a different body part. Chapter 6 describes the application of STR for these muscles of the trunk: rhomboids, pectorals, levator scapulae, upper trapezius, erector spinae and scalenes. Chapter 7 contains stretches for the lower limbs: hamstrings, calf, tensor fasciae latae and the ITB, foot (underside), quadriceps, tibialis anterior, peroneals, gluteals and iliacus. Chapter 8 focuses on the application of STR to these muscles of the upper limbs: triceps, biceps, shoulder adductors, infraspinatus, wrist and finger extensors, and wrist and finger flexors. Illustrations of each of the muscles in these three chapters have been added, along with illustrations showing common trigger points and a description of how STR might be used to address them. References pertaining to the deactivation of trigger points in specific muscles have been included throughout. Arrows have been added to photographs in these chapters, showing in which direction slack in the skin is taken up at the start of the technique. Alternate treatment positions have been added to all chapters.

Chapter 6, Soft Tissue Release for the Trunk, has been improved by the addition of photographs, anatomical illustrations, and new sections on active-assisted STR to rhomboids and pectorals and active STR to trapezius, pectorals and scalenes.

New photographs, anatomical illustrations and sections on passive STR to gluteals, active STR to gluteals and active-assisted STR to the ITB have been added to chapter 7, Soft Tissue Release for the Lower Limbs.

Chapter 8, Soft Tissue Release for the Upper Limbs, has new photographs and illustrations along with new sections on passive STR to shoulder adductors, active STR to shoulder adductors and active-assisted STR to infraspinatus.

Finally, part IV includes a comprehensive chapter on client consultation and designing individualised STR programmes. Two new case studies have been added to this chapter, specifically about the use of STR to deactivate trigger points.

In summary, this edition of *Soft Tissue and Trigger Point Release* contains the following additions:

- 153 new photographs
- 21 anatomical illustrations

- More photographic examples of handholds used to apply locks
- Arrows showing the direction in which to apply pressure to take up slack in soft tissues
- Photographs and text describing variations on treatment positions
- Information about current research on stretching
- A new section on the use of STR to deactivate trigger points
- Illustrations of common trigger points found in each of 21 muscles
- More tips throughout the text
- Overview tables in chapters 3 through 5 with thumbnail photographs showing all of the techniques and positions described in the chapter
- A new section in each chapter with ideas for how to become proficient in the use of that particular form of STR
- A new section describing how to apply passive STR to shoulder adductors
- New sections describing active-assisted STR to the iliotibial band (ITB), infraspinatus, biceps brachii and triceps
- New sections describing how to apply active STR to gluteals, trapezius, scalenes, rhomboid and pectoral muscles

How to Use This Book

You have several different options for using this book to help you become proficient in the application of STR technique.

- *Option 1:* The easiest way might be to use it in conjunction with the continuing education (CE) course and video, in which the technique is demonstrated. Both review questions and exam questions in the CE course will help consolidate your learning.
- *Option 2:* You could learn the technique by choosing to concentrate on one of the three different forms of STR (passive, active-assisted and active), described in chapters 3, 4 and 5.
- *Option 3:* You could practise applying any of the STR variants but focus on one particular part of the body. For example, you could practise working through chapter 7 for the lower limbs.

As you will discover, there are many different ways to apply STR. I hope that you will experiment with them all in order to find the ones that work best for you. Massage therapy is a vibrant, dynamic profession that gains from collaboration and discussion. Feel free to send comments, enquiries and suggestions to me by posting these to The Friendly Physio group on Facebook.

Acknowledgements

It is with grateful thanks that I acknowledge everyone at Human Kinetics who has helped bring this title to print. Decision makers, editors, designers, artists, proofreaders and photographers have each contributed, and as author, I am honoured to be part of this team.

PART I

Getting Started With Soft Tissue Release

This first part of the book provides everything necessary to help you get started with the great technique of soft tissue release (STR).

Chapter 1 teaches you about the kinds of clients for whom STR is appropriate, how the technique works, the kinds of settings in which it can be performed, its benefits and the kinds of conditions for which it is helpful. Here you will also find information about trigger points and how you can utilise STR to help deactivate them. As STR is a stretching technique, this chapter concludes with some research on this topic. Chapter 2 describes how to use your body to apply STR and when the use of tools might be indicated. Also covered in this chapter is the importance of the client consultation, simple safety points and a brief description of the three methods of applying STR. The chapter includes ideas for measuring the effectiveness of STR as well as answers to frequently asked questions and lots of troubleshooting tips, which are useful to refer back to as you work through the book. At the end of these chapters and each subsequent chapter you will discover some quick questions, which you may wish to answer to determine your level of understanding.

Introduction to Soft Tissue Release

Soft tissue release (commonly called STR) is an advanced massage technique widely used in assessing and stretching soft tissues. Soft tissues include muscle fibres, their tendons and the deep and superficial fascia surrounding and invaginating these tissues. Stretching is often used for easing the pain of muscle tension and realigning the body so that it functions in a more optimal way. However, unlike generalised stretching, soft tissue release targets specific areas of tension within a muscle. It is also useful for targeting muscles that are difficult to stretch actively (the fibularis muscle group, or peroneals, for example) and for isolating a muscle within a group of muscles that would normally stretch together (the vastus lateralis from the quadriceps, for example). It has proven useful in the treatment of certain conditions such as medial and lateral epicondylitis and plantar fasciitis, perhaps because it stimulates tissue repair in these conditions.

There are many different forms of stretching. Unlike traditional stretching, STR involves the application of pressure to part of a muscle during the stretch. In this respect, it may be likened to Thai yoga massage. However, unlike Thai yoga massage, it does not target specific acupressure points and is not applied along specific sen lines (meridians; *sen* means 'channel'). When applying STR, pressure is applied either generally (for the purposes of general stretching) or, more commonly, to a specific area of soft tissue that the therapist and client perceive to be tensioned, regardless of whether this happens to fall on a particular acupoint or meridian. The field of STR stretching needs more scientific research; however, the information in this book is based on the author's experience over many years of clinical practice. Stretching in general is believed to be beneficial for overall health, and the American College of Sports Medicine (2018) recommends that stretching is performed 2 to 3 days a week, with each stretch held for 10 to 30 seconds, repeated 2 to 4 times per muscle group, to include the neck, shoulders, trunk, lower back, chest, hips, anterior and posterior legs, and ankles. Because there has been no research into the use of STR as a stretching technique, it is not known whether these guidelines would also apply to STR. STR is almost always performed as part of a massage routine, where massage is used to soothe and stretch tissues following this lock-and-stretch approach; therefore, it is likely that benefits of STR reported by clients and therapists are the result of both the stretch and the massage combined. It is unknown to what extent the individual modalities contribute to achieving the overall treatment outcome.

One of the uses of STR is to help reduce feelings of tension in muscles. It seems logical to therefore use it when a client reports tightness or stiffness. However, a recent study by Stanton et al. (2017) found that participants who reported feeling stiff in the spine did not have a reduced range of motion (mechanical stiffness) of the spine, compared to participants who reported no stiffness. It is not known why this was, but the authors suggested that the participants who reported stiffness overestimated the amount of force being applied to their spine and were better able to detect changes in that force. Interestingly, they then applied the force they were using as different sounds were played. Not surprisingly, when a creaky sound was played, participants reported thinking a higher level of force was being applied compared to when a 'whoosh' sound was played. The authors concluded that feelings of stiffness were not related to actual biomechanical stiffness but may represent a protective construct. In a similar fashion, this raises the question as to whether so-called tight muscles are actually tight. Do people with tight muscles have a reduced range of motion compared to those who do not report tightness? If you have ever treated professional dancers, you will know that they have greater than normal range of motion in the joints compared to the general population and yet still often complain that their muscles feel tight. Does this mean that we should stop stretching people who report back stiffness or tight quadriceps and that stretching is of no benefit to them in feeling less stiff or less tight? No, it means that all forms of stretching, including STR, need to be evaluated in light of ongoing research and that you should determine in advance how you are going to measure the effect of your treatment so that you and your client can decide afterwards whether it was effective. The science of stretching is complex. Until definitive protocols are established, it is likely that different forms of stretching will continue to be of value to different clients.

Who Should Have Soft Tissue Release

Almost anyone will benefit from STR. It is particularly useful for the following people:

- *Anyone who takes part in sports or exercise.* Those taking part in a regular stretching programme will benefit from STR. It is useful before an event when time is limited and the athlete wants to target specific areas of tension; in this case, STR may be applied in a light and brisk manner. Between events it is useful as an assessment tool for identifying tightness in tissues that may limit performance.

- *Anyone recovering from a musculoskeletal injury.* Soft tissues shorten, atrophy and weaken as a result of immobility. Used correctly, STR may help to lengthen and encourage pliability in tight tissues. In this way it helps a client regain range of motion in a joint. Active stretching is known to help with the orientation of collagen fibres during healing.

- *Anyone who maintains a static posture for long periods.* Office workers and drivers who remain seated for long periods often have neck and shoulder pain due to increased muscle tension. STR may be used for alleviating neck pain associated with static postures.

- *Anyone seeking treatment for lateral epicondylitis, medial epicondylitis or plantar fasciitis.* It is also used as an adjunct in the treatment of shin splints and tight hamstrings. Applying STR to the pectorals is helpful for overcoming kyphotic postures.

- *Anyone needing treatment for increased muscle tension and for old scar tissue.* Such areas are palpable, and STR provides the therapist with an additional massage tool to help stretch and realign areas of soft tissue popularly described as being congested.

- *Anyone who needs treatment of trigger points* (localized muscle fibres believed to be in an unhealthy state of contraction and tender to the touch).

How Soft Tissue Release Works

Take a look at the pictures shown in figures 1.1 through 1.3. They represent what happens when a gross stretch is applied to a muscle. The therapist is holding two resistance bands tied together—one red, the other black. The red resistance band is extremely stretchy; the black is tough and less stretchy. The red resistance band represents normal, healthy muscle tissue; the black resistance band represents an area of tight muscle tissue. Together these bands represent one whole muscle. Look at what happens in figure 1.1 when the therapist moves his right hand. Which part of the muscle does the stretching—the pliable (red) part or the tough (black) part? Clearly, the pliable band is doing the most stretching.

Now look at figure 1.2. What happens when the therapist moves his left hand? Which part of the muscle stretches the most—the pliable (red) part or the tough (black) part? Again, the pliable band is doing most of the stretching.

Finally, notice what happens when the therapist moves both his right and left hands apart so they are equidistant (figure 1.3).

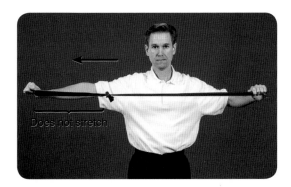

Figure 1.1 Notice which band is doing the stretching.

You can see from the illustrations that the pliable part of the muscle (the red band) does most of the stretching, irrespective of which end of the muscle is moved. To target the less pliable part of the muscle—the area of palpable tightness—you need to localize the stretch. This is exactly what STR does.

To localize the stretch, you need to 'fix' part of the muscle against underlying structures to create a false insertion point. The fixing—described throughout this book as a *lock*—prevents some parts of the muscle from moving and is achieved when a therapist uses his or her own upper body or a massage tool. When a muscle is stretched, its insertion points are moved apart from one another; that is, the area of tissue between the insertion points stretches. Creating false insertion points results in a more intense stretch in some parts of the muscle.

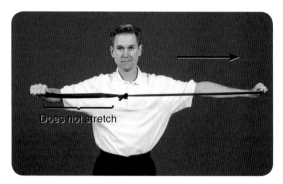

Figure 1.2 Which band is doing the stretching now?

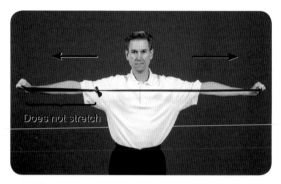

Figure 1.3 Even with an equidistant stretch, the more pliable band does the most stretching.

Look at figure 1.4a, which is an illustration of the soleus. You probably already know that the soleus originates from the posterior shaft of the tibia and inserts into the calcaneus. When resting in the prone position, the foot naturally falls into plantar flexion (figure 1.4b). If you pull up your toes (dorsiflexing your foot and ankle), it stretches the muscles of the calf (which are the plantar flexors). Dorsiflexion is therefore a way of applying a gross stretch to the soleus and may be achieved passively, as illustrated in figure 1.4c.

Now look at figure 1.5a. Imagine locking the muscle to the tibia slightly distal to its actual origin (lock A; figure 1.5b). Can you see that if you were to stretch the muscle now (figure 1.5c), only those fibres running from the new origin (lock A) to the calcaneus would be able to stretch? Would you agree that, providing you are able to dorsiflex through the *same* range of motion as in the first stretch, greater force has been placed on those fibres being stretched? This occurs because the small amount of muscle tissue superior to lock A is no longer being stretched.

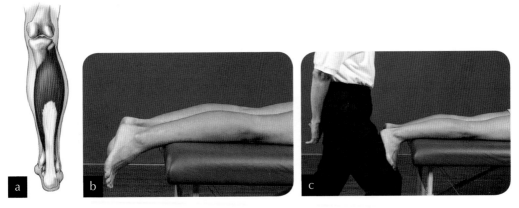

Figure 1.4 *(a)* The soleus; *(b)* the ankle falls into plantar flexion in the prone position; *(c)* performing a passive calf stretch.

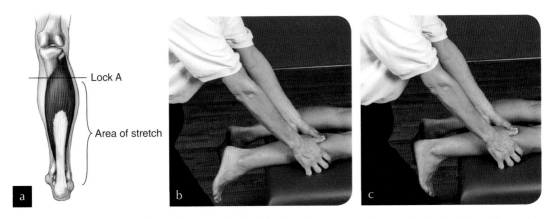

Figure 1.5 *(a)* Locking the soleus muscle slightly distal to its actual origin (lock A); *(b)* applying the lock; *(c)* performing the stretch.

Now look at figure 1.6a. A second imaginary origin (lock B) for the soleus is even more distal on the tibia, broadly locking it to the underlying structures (figure 1.6b). Performing a stretch now (figure 1.6c) will place even greater tension on the stretching fibres than if the lock had remained at lock A.

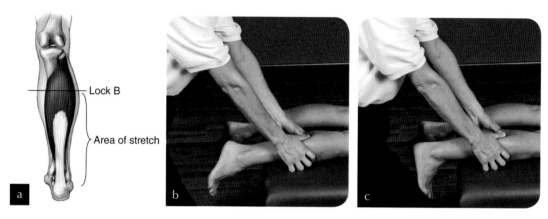

Figure 1.6 (a) Locking the soleus more distal on the tibia (lock B); (b) applying the lock; (c) performing the stretch.

Finally, you could create a third false origin (lock C) yet more distal to the actual origin (see figures 1.7a and 1.7b). In this example, only the most distal portion of the soleus stretches when the foot and ankle are dorsiflexed (figure 1.7c).

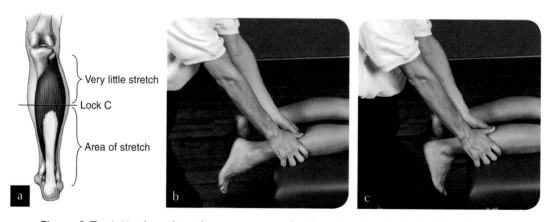

Figure 1.7 (a) Locking the soleus even more distal on the tibia (lock C); (b) applying the lock; (c) performing the stretch.

In reality it is not possible—or advisable—to lock the entire breadth of the muscle, but this is the principle behind how STR works. An alternative is to apply a specific rather than a broad lock—for example, on the biceps brachii, as illustrated in figure 1.8. The areas of muscle fibre distal to each of the locks are put under greater stretch each time the elbow is extended. To understand this concept of a specific stretch, think of muscle fibres as the strings of a guitar. Placing your finger across all of the strings, as in the previous example of the soleus, is quite different from placing your finger across one string, as in the case of using your elbow to apply a lock to the biceps. For a start, it is quite difficult to exert the same pressure across all strings that you would use to fix just one string. When playing the guitar, if you use the tip and pad of your finger to fix just one string, with one specific lock, only that string is affected, yet it is affected intensely. However, if you use more of your finger in an attempt to make a lock across all of the strings, you affect all of the strings when you play, though perhaps not as intensely.

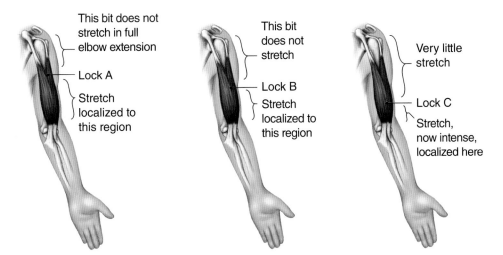

Figure 1.8 In applying specific locks, the areas of muscle fibre distal to each of the locks are put under greater stretch each time the elbow is extended.

Where to Perform Soft Tissue Release

You can use STR anywhere because it may be performed through clothing or a towel and in prone, supine or seated positions.

- *In the office.* When working at a computer or with other office equipment, office workers may find it useful to apply active STR to their wrist and finger flexors and extensors.

- *Whilst seated.* STR can be applied actively to the soles of the feet using a spikey ball or foot roller. STR may also be applied actively to the quadriceps when sitting. Therapists who provide seated, on-site massage may benefit from applying STR to the levator scapulae and the upper trapezius.

- *In the park.* STR to the hamstrings and tibialis anterior can be performed in the park or by the side of a running track.

- *On the tennis court.* After a match, STR to wrist and finger extensors can provide temporary relief from the discomfort of lateral epicondylitis (tennis elbow).

- *On the golf course.* STR may provide temporary relief from medial epicondylitis (golfer's elbow).

- *By the pool.* By working through a towel and taking care to keep the client warm, a therapist may apply STR to all major muscle groups.

- *In the clinic.* STR can be performed as part of a holistic massage treatment, or it could form an entire treatment session in itself. Clinic sessions are useful when working with sensitive areas such as the iliacus because the client needs to be comfortable and relaxed.

- *At home.* Almost anyone can follow a home stretching programme using simple tools to apply a gentle lock into soft tissues.

When to Perform Soft Tissue Release

When performed slowly and conscientiously, soft tissue release may be used before, during or after a massage treatment or as a treatment in itself. Soft tissue becomes more pliable when warm, and most forms of stretching may be more effective when applied to warm tissues. However, increases in joint range are also attainable when STR is applied to tissues that have not been warmed. It is a perfectly safe form of stretching, providing movements are slow and controlled.

Stretching decreases muscle force and should therefore be used with caution in a pre-event setting. In this case it could help increase range of motion in joints, as long as care is taken not to overstretch the associated muscles. It may be valuable in helping to overcome excessive tightness or spasming in localized areas of tissue that need immediate attention before a sporting event.

When using STR in a post-event setting, take care not to work too deeply. There may be microtrauma to tissues, so it is best to use STR conservatively as an assessment tool and save deeper work for part of a maintenance massage. Also, after excessive exercise or training, increased levels of pain-relieving hormones may decrease a client's perception of pain, and as a result, a client may be less able to give accurate feedback relating to the degree of pressure he or she is sensing. In both pre- and post-event work, STR tends to be used as an adjunct to other forms of treatment for overcoming cramping and for maintaining muscle length. Between training sessions and as part of some forms of rehabilitation, it may be used as a form of deep, intense stretching.

Overall, STR should be used when there is a reason to use it. This reason could be simply because the client likes the sensation of STR or because as a therapist you have identified areas of tension that need to be addressed. It is unlikely that you will be working with the same client on a daily basis unless the client is preparing for or involved in an ongoing sporting event. STR can certainly be used weekly, and perhaps two or three times a week, on the same muscle. Use your own judgement to ensure you do not overwork an area. Once STR has been applied two or three times to a muscle within a treatment session, the muscle will be noticeably more pliable.

Benefits of Soft Tissue Release

Soft tissue release is used for a variety of reasons, perhaps most commonly because it stretches soft tissues. It is therefore beneficial because it improves flexibility and posture, alleviates the pain of muscle tension and takes pressure off associated joint structures. It helps maintain or increase range of motion within a joint and, combined with excellent palpation skills, helps therapists assess the degree of tension within and between soft tissues. Many clients also enjoy the sensation of STR and are happy to have it incorporated into their massage routines. It provides therapists with another tool they can employ and may thus help keep massage routines varied. STR is especially useful in clinical settings where clients need to stretch muscles but cannot take joints through a full range of motion. For example, after many forms of knee surgery, patients are encouraged to flex and extend their knees to maintain joint integrity and pliability of surrounding tissue. Movement is believed to facilitate the healing process but is often limited due to pain and

CLIENT TALK

I used STR for the quadriceps of a client who had been in a full-length leg cast and, because of tightening of the knee joint capsule, was initially unable to gain full knee flexion. We started cautiously, gaining very small increases in joint range initially, combining STR with massage in an attempt to stimulate the quadriceps. I had to hold the client's leg in extension and lower it passively because he did not have strength in his quadriceps to do this. I learned that applying passive STR to the quadriceps is actually quite strenuous for the therapist, and I had to take great care not to strain my back whilst performing it.

swelling. Used at the right juncture in treatment, STR can help in stretching the tissues without causing the joint to move through its full range; for example, STR can be applied to the quadriceps with the client flexing the knee to only 90 degrees. STR is particularly useful as part of the rehabilitation process when used for achieving small increases in range that might not otherwise be possible.

Soft Tissue Release and Trigger Points

Myofascial trigger points are specific spots within skeletal muscle that are palpably tensioned and that clients report as being uncomfortable or painful when pressed; they refer pain in a characteristic pattern and may be eliminated with manual therapy. They were described by Simons, Travell and Simons (1999) as 'a hyperirritable spot in skeletal muscle that is associated with a hypersensitive palpable nodule in a taught band' (p.5) and by Leon Chaitow (2000) as 'localized areas of deep tenderness and increased resistance, and digital pressure on such a trigger will often produce twitching and fasciculation' (p.35). Although debate continues within the scientific community as to the presence of trigger points, they are widely acknowledged by manual therapists who report being able to identify them with palpation. Massage and other modalities such as dry needling, anaesthetic injection and cryostretching are reported to reduce the hypersensitivity of these points and thus reduce the pain associated with them. Both massage and stretching are used to deactivate trigger points. As STR combines these methods, it is postulated that STR can be used as a meaningful treatment in its own right. This book guides you in the application of STR to treat trigger points, with illustrations showing common trigger points in the trunk (chapter 6), lower limbs (chapter 7) and upper limbs (chapter 8).

Why You Should Treat Trigger Points

Trigger points are associated with a variety of problems, such as the following:

- Tight and weak muscles
- Decreased muscular strength
- Stiff joints
- Joint pain
- Muscle pain

They have also been associated with headaches, blurred vision, dizziness and sinus problems (Davies, 2004).

How to Identify a Trigger Point

Trigger points emit electrical signals that are measurable. Clinically, they are easily detected because they are located in the belly of the muscle, hurt when pressed firmly, and refer pain in a predictable pattern. If you run your finger or thumb firmly over a muscle containing a trigger point it can be felt as a pea-shaped area of increased tension, and your client will no doubt inform you that you have located it. The muscle here is firm to touch and resistant to pressure and may feel warm. When pressed, tissues elicit what is called a jump sign; that is, when you twang them they produce a characteristic twitch. Another interesting characteristic of trigger points is that they may be latent or active. Simons, Travell and Simons (1999) describe latent trigger points as 'clinically quiescent with respect to spontaneous pain' (p. 4), meaning these points are only painful when pressed. By comparison, an active trigger point 'is always tender' (p. 1) and produces referred pain and tenderness. Both forms of trigger point have a taught band within them that restricts range of motion (p.4).

How You Should Treat Trigger Points

Trigger points may be reduced by the application of gentle pressure. Techniques vary. Davies (2004) suggests stroking the point 6 to 12 times a day. For a client self-treating, this advice is valuable, but for a therapist it is obviously impractical. The use of STR can be beneficial in reducing trigger points, using the following method:

1. Identify the trigger point. Palpate the area and elicit feedback from your client.

2. Follow the guidelines for the application of passive or passive-assisted STR, and passively shorten the muscle in which the trigger point is located, where this is possible.

3. Apply gentle pressure. On a scale of 0 to 10, with 10 being worst pain ever and 0 being no pain at all, ask your client to inform you how painful the pressure is that you are applying. Whilst many therapists use a level 7 pain as a guide when treating trigger points, the author recommends working at around a level 5. The rationale for this approach is twofold. Firstly, as soft issues are lengthened and stretched with STR, tension increases naturally and pain can increase. Secondly, increased pain causes more muscle tension or muscle guarding by the patient, which is counterproductive to reducing trigger points.

4. Following the guidelines for the application of STR to whichever muscle you are treating (which can be found in chapters 6, 7 and 8 of this book), gently stretch the muscle using STR and then soothe the area with massage.

5. Relocate the trigger point, apply gentle pressure, and ask your client to inform you whether the same level of pressure elicits the same level of pain. If the use of STR has been successful, your client should report that he or she feels less pain when you apply the same degree of pressure as previously. You can repeat the technique a second time if necessary. Often releasing a trigger will increase joint range of motion and muscle extensibility.

Closing Remarks

You have learned that soft tissue release targets specific areas of tension in a muscle. It especially stretches the muscle fibres, their tendons and the fascia. It is safe and effective for most people.

Now that you have an idea of what STR is, how it works, who could receive it and when and where you can use it, you are ready to discover more about the various ways of locking muscles and using massage tools. In addition, you are ready to learn lots of tips and tricks for using this technique as well as ideas for measuring your effectiveness.

Quick Questions

1. How does STR differ from generalised stretching?
2. Give three examples of how a muscle might be locked.
3. When applying a lock, do you start at the proximal or distal end of the muscle?
4. Why should STR be used cautiously in a pre-event setting?
5. Why should deep STR be avoided in a post-event setting?
6. Give three examples of the kinds of muscular problems associated with trigger points.
7. Give two examples of the kinds of joint problems associated with trigger points.

Preparing for Soft Tissue Release

In this chapter, you will learn the following basics of STR: various methods of locking tissues, including their advantages and disadvantages; using massage tools to apply STR; potential safety issues; and an overview of the three types of STR—passive, active-assisted and active. At the end of the chapter, you'll find frequently asked questions and troubleshooting tips, as well as a section on measuring the effectiveness of your treatments. After completing the chapter, you will have everything you need to get started with this versatile stretching technique.

Using Your Body to Apply STR

STR may be applied without any equipment at all. In a later section, you'll read about using tools to help lock muscles. This section explains how your upper body provides an array of options for applying STR. Forearms can provide broad locks, and elbows can provide localized locks; similarly, you can use each part of the upper limb for unique purposes. Massage therapists are notorious for sustaining upper limb injuries due to overuse. You can easily avoid these injuries by using your forearms, fists and elbows as described in the following text and photos.

Forearm

Forearms are used on large, bulky muscles, such as the calf (a and b), hamstrings (c), quadriceps (d) and gluteals (e). They can also be used when working on the upper fibres of the trapezius (f), using less pressure than when working on the lower limbs. Your forearm provides a strong, broad lock, good for providing overall stretch and for use with clients who cannot tolerate a more specific lock. These locks are easy to apply. The amount of contact with the client's muscles can be varied; for example, a forearm lock to the quadriceps is broad, whereas a lock to the calf is a little more specific. Even though forearm locks create more leverage and are safer for the therapist's own joints, some therapists avoid these locks, claiming they find it difficult to assess tissues without using their hands. It is worth practicing STR using your forearms in order to avoid potential overuse injuries. The disadvantage of using your forearms is that they provide a less specific stretch than your elbow does, and forearms are difficult to use on small muscle groups.

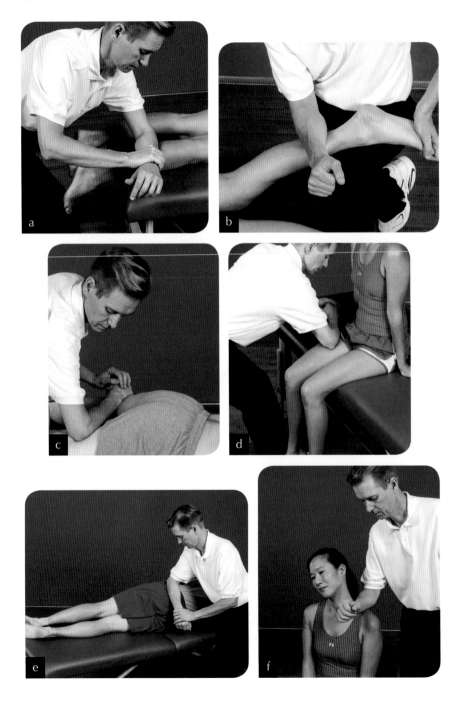

Elbow

Elbows are used in applying firm, deep pressure, which locks tissues in such a way as to direct the stretch to the tight parts of the muscle. Elbows are good for working large, bulky muscles as when treating clients with well-developed calves (a), especially when a client wants to stretch a muscle actively or where palpable tightness exists, perhaps resulting from scar tissue. Elbows are also useful for targeting strap-like muscles, such as the levator scapulae (b), or on muscles that would not be properly locked with the use of forearms due to their location, such as tibialis anterior (c) and fibularis (peroneal) muscles. Using an elbow to lock tissues does not necessitate the application of force. With practice, elbows may be used sensitively on levator scapulae and around the upper fibres of the trapezius in order to provide a localized lock. As with the finger or thumb, the elbow provides such a specific lock that it can be used to apply STR to help deactivate trigger points once they have been identified through palpation.

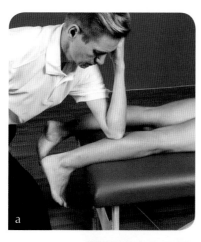
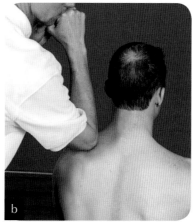
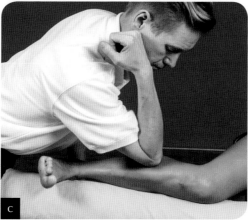

Single Fist

Sometimes it is necessary to provide a broad lock, but there is not enough room for your forearm or hands. To work an area more specifically than with a forearm but less specifically than with an elbow, you could use a single fist. Using cupped fingers and applying a soft fist works well on pectorals (*a, b* and *c*), hamstrings (*d*), biceps (*e*) and even tibialis anterior (*f*) when working with a client in the prone position. Notice from these photographs how, when using your fist to apply STR to the pectorals, the client's arm can be held in various different positions (*a* and *b*) to suit your preferred application of the technique.

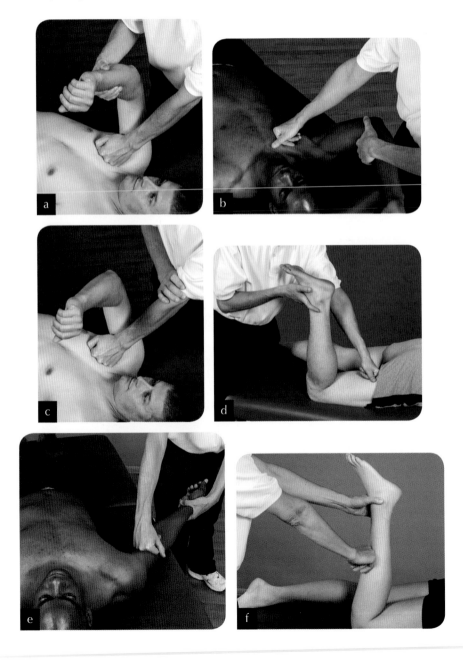

Double Fist

Where firm pressure is required, use of a double fist can be helpful, cupping one fist inside the other as in the photograph of STR to the iliotibial band (ITB; *a*) on the side of the thigh. However, you can use fists side-by-side to provide a softer lock, as when working on the calf with your client in either the prone position (*b*) or side-lying position (*c*).

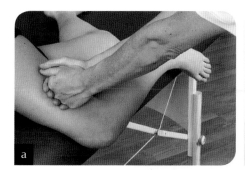
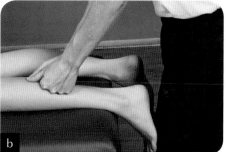

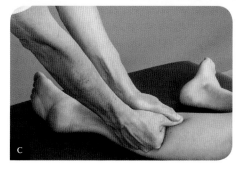

Palm

Palms provide a flat surface for a lock but place some stress on the therapist's wrist joint, so you should use them with care. Because palm pressure is not deep, it is good for providing a gentle lock, which is useful for the application of mild STR before or after sporting events, for example. Use of the palm as a lock can be helpful when working latissimus dorsi (*a*) and the tissues around the armpit (*b*), with your client in either the prone position or the side-lying position.

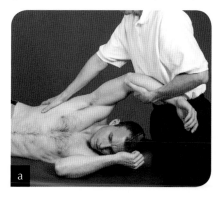
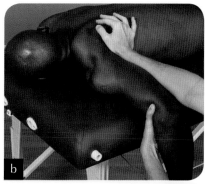

Gripping and Squeezing

Sometimes simply gripping the muscle can be a way of providing a lock. Gripping works best on small biceps and triceps (a) that do not require a great degree of stretch. To avoid pinching the muscle, simply apply some oil and grip through a facecloth or small towel. Another use of this type of lock is as a squeezing motion to the calf when the client is in the prone position (b).

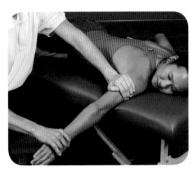
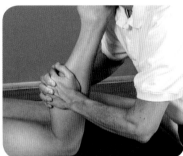

Reinforced Thumbs

Reinforced thumbs are used in locking specific areas of muscle, generally smaller muscles that do not require much force for a lock. They work well on the common flexor (a) and extensor (b) origins of the wrist, and the fibulari (c). You can use reinforced thumbs even when working on the calf (d), but take care as this stronger muscle usually requires the force of a stronger lock. If you discover that you need to apply a lot of pressure through your thumbs, then change the form of lock you are using. Practise applying gentle pressure through your forearms or elbow rather than risk damaging your thumb joints. It may necessitate working with the client in a seated position.

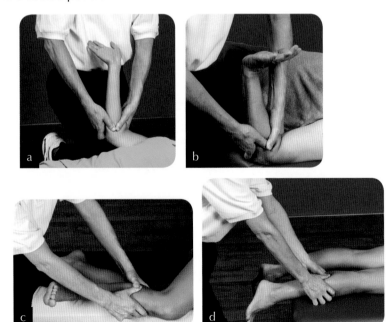

Single Thumb

Thumbs must be used with caution and only to lock tissues when gentle pressure is required; for example, when working on the biceps (a), wrist flexors (b) and wrist extensors (c). The thumb can be helpful in identifying levator scapulae (d) prior to the application of a deeper lock using an elbow, for example; but when this area is tender and only light pressure is required, you can use the thumb here, too. You can use the thumb when applying STR to the rhomboids with the client in a seated position (e). However, in so doing, it is used to take up slack in the skin, pushing it gently toward the spine rather than using it to place downwards pressure into the rhomboids. In such cases, it is not as effective as when working with a client in the prone position, but it can help when treating a client who cannot rest prone, or when applying STR to help eliminate trigger points. Overuse of thumbs during treatment is a common cause of injury for massage therapists. Wherever possible, use an alternative method of locking.

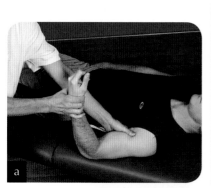
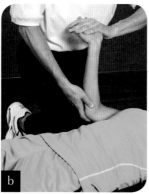
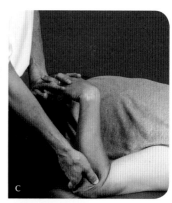
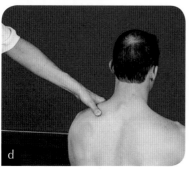
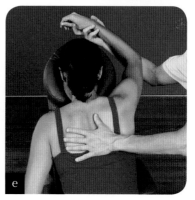

Fingers

It is useful to use fingers to lock sensitive tissues, such as the scalene muscles (a), that require very little pressure, with your client either seated or in the supine position. You may also use fingers to apply gentle STR to the upper part of the chest when working with a client for whom very little pressure is needed (b), or where the chest area is small. Fingers may also be useful in applying STR to the iliacus, and you may cup them for reinforcement (c).

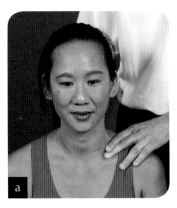
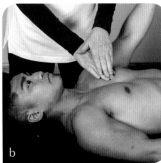
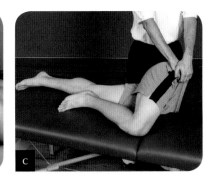

Knuckles

Knuckles are useful for applying a lock to erector spinae muscles with your client seated and are a good alternative to thumbs. As with the application of all forms of STR, it is important to keep your knuckle lock static. Avoid *worrying* the tissues (rubbing in a manner that causes friction), because it simply grinds your knuckle joints.

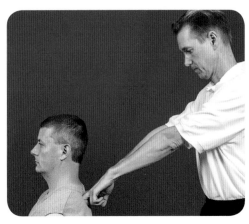

Using knuckles to erector spinae.

Using Tools to Apply STR

As with the application of all forms of therapy, you need to protect your own body when working. Fortunately, you can apply STR safely and effectively if you follow certain guidelines, and a variety of tools provide additional support. Shown here is a selection of tools designed for use in bodywork as well as some objects that have been improvised for this purpose.

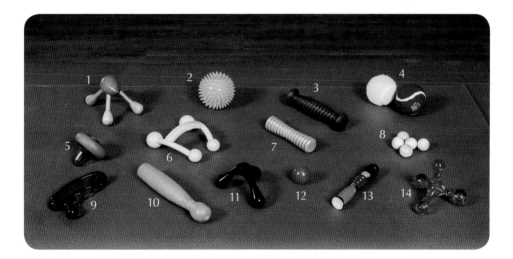

1. Wooden 'mouse'
2. Plastic therapy ball with spikes
3. Wooden foot roller (convex)
4. Tennis-type balls from a pet shop
5. The Knobble massage tool
6. Hard plastic Quad Nobber
7. Wooden foot roller (concave), also used on forearms
8. Wooden spheres from a hardware store
9. Index Knobber
10. Child's wooden skittle from a thrift shop
11. Hard plastic massage tool
12. Plastic high-bounce ball (soft) from a toy shop
13. Child's wooden toy soldier
14. Plastic Jacknobber

Shown here is an Index Knobber being used in treating the sole of the foot. It could work equally well on any area that required deep, localized pressure; it makes a good alternative to using your thumb, as does the Jacknobber, shown here being applied to the sole of the foot with the client in the supine position.

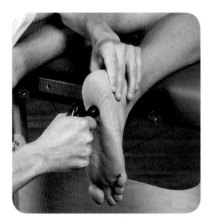

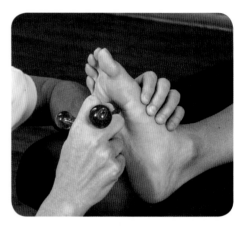

Index Knobber to sole of foot with client in the prone position.

Jacknobber to sole of foot with client in the supine position.

The spikey therapy balls are useful for applying active STR to the soles of the feet when sitting.

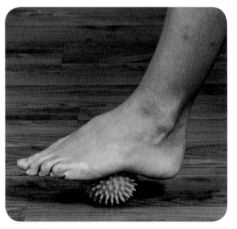

Spikey ball to sole of foot.

The tennis-type balls are actually for dogs and deform much less readily than regular tennis balls. They are useful for applying active STR to hamstrings or quadriceps, as shown here.

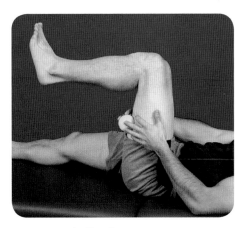

Tennis-type ball to hamstrings.

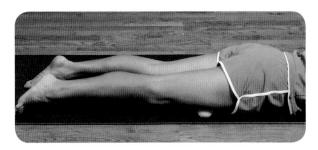

Tennis-type ball to quadriceps.

Both an Index Knobber and tennis-type ball can be useful for active-assisted STR to the upper trapezius, as shown in the following photographs.

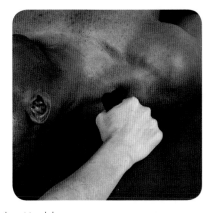
Index Knobber to upper trapezius.

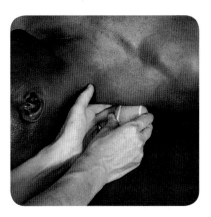
Tennis-type ball to upper trapezius.

Other pieces of useful equipment include a facecloth or small towel and some massage oil. STR can be applied through clothing, but for a stronger lock, apply oil to the client's skin and work through a facecloth or small towel.

Consultation With the Client

As with all forms of therapy, when you meet a client for the first time, start with an initial client consultation in which you discover the nature of your client's problem and what he or she hopes to gain from your treatment. Take a detailed history, making note of any medication the client is taking, and identify any con-traindications to your treatment plan. Then carry out a physical assessment, which will vary depending on what it is you will be treating. For example, in assessing someone who has come to you because he or she still has a stiff joint from an old ankle sprain, you will need to test the ankle's range of motion; if you are dealing with an office worker who has neck pain, you may want to do a seated postural assessment of the upper body.

When using STR to help deactivate trigger points, establish how your client is going to feed back to you with regards to their level of discomfort. Remember, trigger points are uncomfortable—even painful—when pressed, so it is important to determine how you will gauge this response. Recall from chapter 1 that many therapists like to imagine that 10 is a number used for describing severe pain, and zero for describing no pain. Using a 0 to 10 pain scale, advise your client to alert you if discomfort exceeds a level 5. Remember to err on the side of caution, at least initially, advising your client that discomfort should not exceed a level 5. Many clients enjoy the sensation of deep tissue massage, and some believe that suffering discomfort is beneficial and a worthwhile means to an end if it reduces feelings of muscle soreness or stiffness. Pain is counterproductive to relaxation. Any client in pain when receiving STR is not likely to benefit, as trigger points are unlikely to be treated effectively when your client is unable to relax.

At the end of your consultation, you will likely set out the aims of your treat-ment (e.g., to alleviate pain, increase range of motion, reduce the sensation of muscle stiffness following exercise), if necessary describing these aims in lay terms to ensure your client is in agreement with what you plan to do and hope to achieve. Chapter 9 covers the topic of client consultation in detail, with sug-gested questions, possible physical assessments and methods of documentation.

Caution and Safety Issues

Soft tissue release is a form of assisted stretching that is safe and effective for the majority of clients. Use this one simple rule to decide whether or not a client may receive soft tissue release: If you would not normally treat the client with massage, bodywork or stretching, the client should not receive STR.

Because the technique involves gentle pressure into soft tissue, exercise caution when applying it to clients who bruise easily or who have thin skin. When treating clients who are hypermobile (increased range of motion in the joints, common amongst professional dancers, for example) consider whether stretching the tissues, and thus improving joint range, is actually desirable. Soft tissue release is not suitable for clients with hypermobility syndromes because the clients already have excessive pliability of tissues.

When first receiving a lock, most clients feel no stretch at all. It is not until the lock nears the distal end of the muscle that the stretch intensifies. If you happen to lock a trigger spot, the client will report slight discomfort. This discomfort should be expressed in terms of being 'comfortably tolerable' or 'it hurts, but it feels good'. If you are a massage therapist, you are probably familiar with such statements. However, if the client reports that the sensation has become truly uncomfortable, you should not perform STR. It may be that there is some underlying inflammation not yet palpable. A general rule is that the feeling of increased localized tension should dissipate within about a minute of applying a lock. If it does not, remove the lock. This feeling is quite unlike that of old scar tissue, which is palpably tight but causes no discomfort.

Although rare, clients sometimes report feeling sore after STR, as with some other forms of stretching. The feeling has been likened to delayed onset muscle soreness (DOMS). For this reason, you should avoid overworking any one particular area and aim to incorporate STR with oil massage if possible. Theoretically, massage between sessions of STR helps flush fresh blood into tissues and improve muscle health. Some therapists like to warn clients that in rare cases soreness may occur but will resolve itself within about 12 hours. However, others argue that this statement sets up a self-fulfilling prophecy and promotes the likelihood that the client will experience that exact soreness.

Pre- and post-event STR should not be applied too deeply. Before an event, it could decrease muscle power and may also be deeply relaxing. Pre-event STR should be used in an upbeat manner and with the aim of invigorating the client and maintaining joint range of motion. Post-event STR may increase the likelihood of bruising after microtrauma to tissues. Post-event STR should be used generally and to help overcome cramping.

As a therapist, you should avoid overusing your upper limbs when applying any technique, including STR. Wherever possible, transfer your body weight through your forearms and elbows or use a massage tool as an alternative to using your thumbs. Save your thumbs and fingers for delicate work on smaller, more pliable tissues. To get even more leverage, try working with your treatment couch an inch or two lower than you have it at present. Practise leaning in to your client, transferring your weight to his or her tissues. Many therapists adopt the position of leaning in but actually use a lot of energy holding the leaning-in stance because they are fearful of hurting the client. Make it your intention to create locks by gently but firmly leaning in towards your client *before* beginning treatment. By working slowly and conscientiously, you will discover that with practice, STR is a powerful, safe and effective tool for stretching soft tissues.

Three Methods of STR

The three ways of performing STR are passive, active-assisted and active (see the examples from Using Wrist Flexors to Compare the Three Types of STR on the next page). They are defined as follows:

1. *Passive.* When STR is performed passively, the therapist applies a lock and moves the client's body part to facilitate a stretch.

2. *Active-assisted.* This form of STR requires the client and therapist to work together. Usually, the therapist applies a lock, and the client moves his or her body part to bring about the stretch.

3. *Active.* In active STR, the client applies a lock to himself or herself and also performs the stretch without assistance. Almost anyone can perform active STR, and the presence of a therapist is not required.

This book uses common anatomical language. However, clients are unlikely to understand these terms unless they are therapists or health professionals themselves. It takes practice to explain to clients what they are required to do for active-assisted STR without using technical language. Many clients may not understand what you mean if you ask them to invert or evert a foot, for example, or to flex or extend a wrist. One tip is to demonstrate the action you require before making your lock. If you want to give the command of 'up' or 'down' when referring to a wrist movement, for example, then you need to demonstrate what you mean by those commands. Another tip is to avoid mixing different types of STR within the same treatment. If you start with active-assisted STR, a client may think he or she is required to assist throughout a treatment and may not relax when you want to perform passive STR. However, many clients soon become accustomed to STR and will demonstrate a preference for whether they want to take part (active assisted) or whether they prefer to receive the treatment passively.

Measuring the Effectiveness of STR

It is useful to have a benchmark against which to measure whether a treatment has been effective. This is equally true of STR. Here are some ideas to help you measure the effectiveness of STR.

■ *Pain.* If STR is being used to alleviate the discomfort of muscle tension, one of the easiest methods for measuring effectiveness is simply to use self-reporting measures. Not surprisingly, most clients feel better after massage and report feeling less discomfort, whether this was initially described as pain, pulling, cramping or aching. Most therapists are familiar with asking clients how they feel after treatment.

■ *Visual analogue scale (VAS).* This scale is simply a horizontal line onto which two extremes have been written (figure 2.1). One extreme could be 'no discomfort' and the other extreme could be 'worst discomfort ever.' Before and after treatment, ask the client to mark the scale according to how he or she is feeling. A VAS is useful for measuring subjective descriptors such as pain or stiffness.

Using Wrist Flexors to Compare the Three Types of STR

PASSIVE STR. The therapist locks the common flexor origin with the client's wrist in flexion and then moves the wrist into extension.

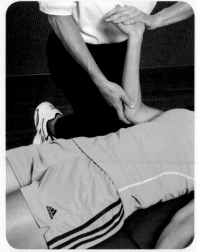

ACTIVE-ASSISTED STR. The therapist locks the client's common flexor origin and then asks the client to extend the wrist actively.

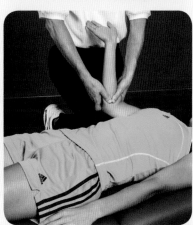

ACTIVE STR. The client locks her own common flexor origin and then extends the wrist.

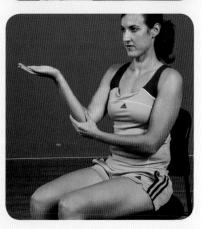

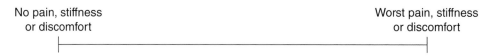

No pain, stiffness   Worst pain, stiffness

or discomfort   or discomfort

Figure 2.1   Visual analogue scale (VAS).

■   *Movement and muscle length tests.* If STR has been applied to help increase range of motion in a joint, you could do tests such as the straight-leg raise for hamstring length (figure 2.2). Measure the straight-leg raise before and after applying STR to the hamstrings, and record whether any increase in range at the hip joint has occurred as a result of your treatment. A simple test for quadriceps flexibility is the prone knee bend (figure 2.3). Ask the client to flex his or her knee whilst in a prone position; observe how close the client's foot comes to the buttock on that side. After treatment to lengthen the quadriceps, the client should be able to reach his or her foot closer to the buttock than before treatment. Make sure the client avoids excessive lordosis in the lower back.

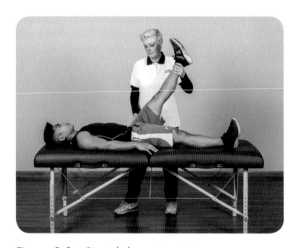

Figure 2.2   Straight-leg raise test.

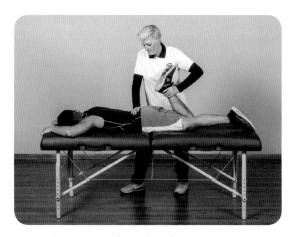

Figure 2.3   Prone knee bend test.

- *Sit-and-reach test.* A simple way to measure the effectiveness of active STR to the hamstrings is to ask your client to reach forward and try to touch his or her toes (figure 2.4). Notice how far the client can reach, and ask what sensations are felt in the hamstring muscles. If you have a tape measure, document how far they can reach with respect to their feet. Spend 5 to 7 minutes applying STR to the hamstrings, then retest the client. Was the client able to touch the toes more easily? Did the client have less tightness in the hamstring muscles? This test also tests flexibility in the muscles of the back and should not be performed by clients who have recently suffered trauma to the lumbar spine.

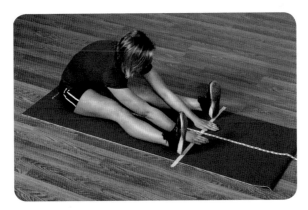

Figure 2.4 Sit-and-reach test.

Frequently Asked Questions and Troubleshooting Tips

How long should I hold my lock at the end of the stretch?

Once the tissues are stretched, remove the lock.

How much pressure should I apply when locking in?

Enough to lock the tissues. If it causes discomfort to the client or to you, read the troubleshooting tips that follow these questions.

Should I encourage the client to tolerate pain?

Never. STR should be comfortable. Clients should feel a mild stretch, but the sensation may vary depending on which part of the muscle you are working.

How many times should I perform STR on one muscle?

You may find that for large muscles, such as hamstrings, you need to work all over them in lines, from proximal to distal, to cover the tissues adequately. Once you have done each line three times, both you and the client should sense that the tissues have stretched. Overall, you need to avoid overworking one muscle group. Sometimes it is a good idea to apply STR two or three times, move to a different part of the body, then return to the original STR site and check to see whether both you and the client perceive the tissue to have stretched.

If after working through this book you are still having difficulty applying STR, here are some things you can try:

- If you can't seem to get a grip on the soft tissue, practise changing your lock. Have you tried using the flat of your palm or a soft fist, forearm, elbow or knuckles? An alternative is to apply a small amount of oil onto the skin, then work through a towel. The towel will grip the oil and provide a stronger lock.

- If the lock is uncomfortable for the client, try using less pressure. Try working through clothing or a small towel to dissipate your lock. Alternatively, make sure you are not putting pressure on bone. It is a common mistake people make when first learning to apply STR to the rhomboids; avoid pressing into the medial border of the scapulae. When working the pectorals, avoid pressing perpendicularly into the ribs. Check that you are not pressing into a nerve plexus, which can cause a tingling sensation for the client. Check that you are not pulling on the skin too hard.

- If your client does not seem to feel the stretch, try adding more pressure. To increase pressure, use your elbows or forearms and lean into the lock. Alternatively, make sure you take up the slack in the soft tissues before performing the stretch. Check that you are directing your pressure towards the proximal end of the limb. Many clients do not experience much of a stretch with passive STR. In this case, try using active STR and see what happens.

- If it is uncomfortable for you to apply the lock with your fingers, hands or thumbs, try using a massage tool. Always aim to protect your own joints. If you still can't apply the lock comfortably, don't do it at all.

- If you can't seem to get comfortable yourself, try changing how you hold the client, altering the height of your couch or adjusting the position of your client on the couch or chair.

- If you are still having difficulty after trying various ways to apply STR, stop using that particular stretch.

Closing Remarks

This chapter has shown the advantages and disadvantages of using different types of locks and considered how and when to use massage tools. The section on commonly asked questions and troubleshooting tips, plus information concerning safety issues and how to measure the effectiveness of STR has helped provide the foundation for using this technique. Now you are ready to practise the three different forms of STR.

Quick Questions

1. Give an example of when you might use your palm to lock tissues.
2. Give examples of three kinds of clients for whom STR is not appropriate.
3. List the three types of STR.
4. For how long do you hold a lock at the end of a stretch?
5. List three ways you could measure the effectiveness of STR.

Soft Tissue Release Techniques

In this part of the book, you will find information on how to apply each of the three types of STR: passive (chapter 3), active-assisted (chapter 4) and active (chapter 5). Each of the three chapters in part II follows the same format: First is a step-by-step description of how to perform the technique. Next, detailed descriptions explain the direction in which to apply locks, how to focus the stretch to a particular area, the direction in which to apply pressure, how to take up slack in the skin and how to incorporate STR with oil massage. Chapter 5 additionally has a section on using active STR as part of a home care programme. Key holds, moves and stances are described, using plenty of examples involving different muscles. This section provides condensed instructions and photos showing the start and end positions of stretches for each muscle. It is important to safeguard yourself and your clients when working, and each chapter therefore contains useful safety guidelines specific to the type of STR being described and when that particular form of STR is indicated. Each chapter also contains a section describing how to use that form of STR to treat trigger points and one on how to become proficient in STR. At the very end of each chapter you will find a table of thumbnail photographs of each of the muscles for which STR has been described. You can use it when practicing the techniques, making notes as to what you have found easy and on which muscles and with which form of STR you need more practice.

When performing STR, remember that some muscles are not usually shortened during the application. This is because it would be technically difficult to lock them once they have been placed in a shortened position. Table 4.1 lists those muscles that are usually shortened and those that are not.

Reading through these chapters will provide you with a clear understanding of the differences among the three types of STR. You will then be ready to practice their application on different parts of the body, as described in chapters 6 to 8.

Passive Soft Tissue Release

In this chapter you will discover how to perform passive STR by working through seven simple steps. To get you started with using this form of the technique, the chapter includes photographs and brief descriptions demonstrating key holds, moves and stances for a variety of muscles, an overview of which is presented in table 3.2 at the end of the chapter; you can also use the table as a checklist when practicing passive STR. Safety guidelines and a table (3.1) illustrate when passive STR may be indicated. Reading this chapter and answering the Quick Questions will give you a good understanding of how passive STR is applied.

Introduction to Passive Soft Tissue Release

Passive soft tissue release is an excellent method of stretching that may be used as a stand-alone technique through clothing or incorporated into a holistic massage. In this form of STR, the therapist shortens a muscle, locks it and then stretches it. The client remains passive throughout but of course may provide feedback regarding the intensity of the stretch.

How to Perform Passive STR

To perform passive STR, follow these steps:

1. *Identify the muscle to be stretched and the direction of the muscle fibres.*
2. *Ensure the muscle is in a neutral position.* Neutral means that the muscle is neither shortened too much nor stretched. Usually, it requires the therapist to passively shorten the muscle.

Some muscles (especially hamstrings) are prone to cramp when shortened. The likelihood of cramping increases after exercise. It is therefore sometimes a good idea to incorporate STR with oil massage, thus aiding the relaxation of muscle fibres, decreasing the likelihood of cramping when these muscles are shortened.

3. *Explain the procedure to the client.* Tell the client that you will be performing the stretch and all he or she needs to do is relax. The muscle on which you are working should be relaxed.

   Gently shaking a limb encourages muscle relaxation and is useful when working with clients who find it difficult to 'switch off' and relax.

4. *Whilst keeping the muscle in the neutral position, gently lock the muscle to fix the fibres.* (See chapter 2 for a variety of locking methods.) Start proximally, nearest to the origin of the muscle. Examples in which locking does not need to begin at the proximal end of the muscle include cases where you can use STR to glide along the muscle distally to proximally, whilst passively moving the joint associated with that muscle. You can find more details about this less common but very useful application at the end of this chapter and in chapter four, and again in chapters seven and eight.

TIP Generally, the origin of the muscle is that part closest to the midline of the body and least movable. Usually, when a muscle contracts, the insertion moves closer to the origin.

5. *Whilst maintaining your lock, stretch the muscle.* Move the body part in such a way that the muscle goes from a shortened to a lengthened position. For example, if you needed to flex a joint to shorten the muscle, you will need to extend the joint to stretch it.

6. *Once the muscle has been stretched, release your lock and return the muscle to neutral.*

7. *Choose another point to fix the muscle, working proximally to distally.* Repeat steps 4 to 6 until you reach the distal tendons of the muscle.

   To really focus your stretch on a particular area, place your locks close together, perhaps a centimeter (0.39 in.) apart, as you work from proximal to distal on a muscle. For a more general, less localised stretch, place your locks 3 to 4 centimetres (1.18-1.57 in.) apart.

Get feedback from your client. Some clients do not feel much of a stretch, simply the pressure of the lock. If you are applying the technique correctly, the stretch will increase as you work on the more distal aspects of the muscle. Stop if the client reports pain.

The Direction of Locks

You may be wondering, How do I know in which direction I should work on a muscle when using passive STR? If treating the calf, for example, do I work from knee to ankle or ankle to knee? Or across the belly of the muscle?

Chapter 1 stated that STR is applied by working proximally to distally on a muscle (figure 3.1*a*). This method is the easiest way for you to apply passive STR and the most comfortable for the client. When applying STR, the stretch will always feel more intense as you work proximally to distally unless you happen to have placed your lock over a trigger point. If you start distally (figure 3.1*b*), the stretch will already be intense, it is hard to apply STR when working in this direction and it can be quite uncomfortable for the client. This chapter introduces a variant of passive STR, a form of gliding STR. Strangely, when using gliding STR it is easiest to work distally to proximally (figure 3.1*c*). Gliding STR works in this manner because it does not involve a series of single, distinguishable locks. Instead, it is applied using a massage medium using a slow, single, firm glide as the joint associated with that muscle is moved. It is comfortable to receive and easy to apply.

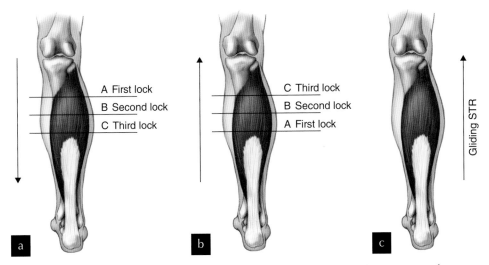

Figure 3.1 It is easiest to apply locks working from the origin to the insertion of a muscle *(a)*, whereas it is more difficult to work from the insertion to the origin *(b)* unless gliding STR is used *(c)*.

When working on long muscles such as the calf, hamstrings, biceps brachii, triceps and muscles of the forearm, you can apply STR by creating a series of separate locks performed one after the other as described in chapter 1, working proximally to distally or, by gliding along the muscle in a very slow, continuous movement working distally to proximally. However, when working muscles such as the rhomboids, pectoralis major or the gluteals, you may find that the area in which you need to lock is small or that the shape of the muscle prevents you working in either of these ways. In such cases you simply work over the area you have, getting feedback from your client as to which lock position provides the greatest stretch.

How to Focus the Stretch to One Area

In chapter 1, figures 1.5, 1.6 and 1.7 illustrate how, as you work proximally to distally down the length of a muscle, the sensation of stretch increases from least to greatest. Figure 3.2 illustrates this concept, showing the application of a broad lock first at point A, then at point B and last, at point C, using the forearm, for example. Compare it to figure 3.3, which illustrates the application of locks close together; they are not only together but would be applied using a more localised lock such as the thumb or elbow. Can you see how applying locks close together will create greater stretch to a localised area than applying locks that are spread across the length of the muscle?

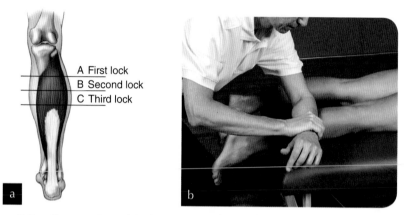

Figure 3.2   Creating broad locks spanning the width of the muscle (a) which, when applied, (b) create a stretch that increases in intensity from point A to point C.

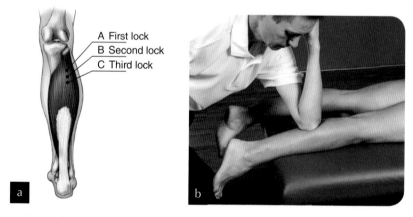

Figure 3.3   Placing locks close together (a) helps focus the stretch to one particular area of muscle (b).

Be aware that whilst it is possible to use STR to focus the stretch to one specific area of muscle, and many therapists use it for this purpose, it is important to always soothe the area with effleurage after using the technique in this way. This approach reduces the likelihood of any soreness.

The Direction of Pressure

The direction to which you apply pressure when placing your lock makes a difference to where your client senses the stretch, the effectiveness of the stretch and how easy it is for you to apply the stretch. Subtle changes in the direction of pressure can make a difference to the effect of this technique. With practice, you will discover that as you passively stretch a client's muscle, the part of your body that you are using to apply the lock gets 'dragged' in a particular direction. It is therefore necessary to counter this movement by applying pressure *opposite* to the direction of drag.

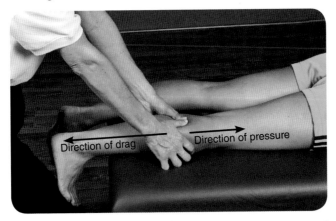

Figure 3.4 The direction of drag is towards the foot when working on the calf, so pressure needs to be directed towards the knee.

For example, when using STR on the calf the direction of drag is towards the foot, so you need to apply pressure towards the knee (figure 3.4). When using STR on the hamstrings, the direction of drag is towards the knee, so you need to apply pressure towards the buttock (figure 3.5).

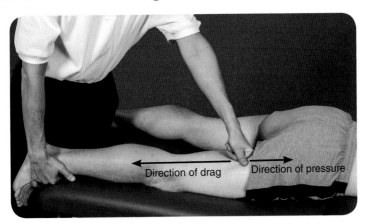

Figure 3.5 Working on the hamstrings the direction of drag towards the knee is countered by directing pressure toward the buttock.

TIP To understand how the direction of pressure affects the application of passive STR, try this exercise: Select a muscle such as the calf, apply your lock pressure perpendicular to the calf and then apply the stretch. Compare it to what happens when you take up some slack in the skin, applying pressure towards the knee. Finally, compare what happens when you apply pressure by pulling the skin of the calf slightly towards you. You (and your client) should sense that the strongest stretch occurs when pressure is directed towards the knee.

Each of the photographs in the section of this chapter called Key Holds, Moves and Stances for Passive Soft Tissue Release have an arrow showing the direction in which you should attempt to direct your pressure.

Taking Up Slack in the Skin

One reason for applying pressure in a particular direction is to take up slack in the skin prior to performing the stretch, as it makes the stretch more effective. Whilst this can readily be felt, it is difficult to illustrate. However, you may get some idea of what is meant by 'take up the slack' from these photographs showing how a therapist might use a thumb to gently push away the skin overlying the lower portion of the trapezius muscle and the rhomboids.

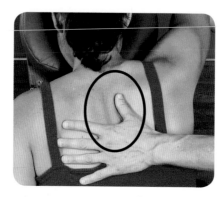

Preparing to take up slack in the skin overlying the rhomboids.

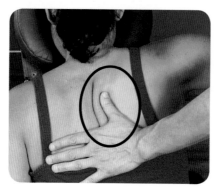

Taking up slack in the skin overlying the rhomboids.

Incorporating STR With Oil Massage

STR is easy to incorporate with oil massage. After the application of oil or massage wax, put a thin towel or facecloth over the area and apply STR through it. Be aware that working this way provides a much stronger lock than working through clothing or on bare skin because the fronds of the fabric grip the massage medium. Remove the towel, clear the area with more massage and repeat. You will discover that if you do this three times (i.e., massage, STR; massage, STR; massage, STR), on your third application of STR, your client will sense less of a stretch (and you will sense less resistance in tissues) because there will be a decrease in tone in the soft tissues after your first two applications.

Another way to incorporate STR with oil or another massage medium is to modify the technique into a gliding technique. For example, when gliding on the calf (a), passively flex and extend the client's ankle; when working on the biceps brachii (b), passively flex and extend the elbow; when treating the wrist and finger extensors (c), passively flex and extend the wrist.

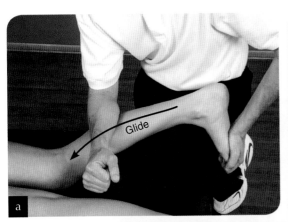
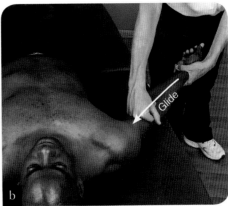
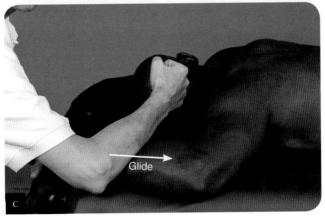

Key Holds, Moves and Stances for Passive STR

This section illustrates these nine areas of the body that lend themselves to passive STR: the calf, hamstrings, gluteals, rhomboids, triceps, biceps, wrist and finger flexors and extensors, and pectorals. Remember that for each of the examples provided here, you need to maintain the gentle pressure of your lock as you passively stretch the tissues. Each photograph includes an arrow showing the direction to which you apply pressure and take up slack in the skin. You can find detailed instructions for these stretches in chapters 6 to 8, where you can compare them to the instructions for active-assisted and active techniques.

Calf

Stand at the end of the couch with your client in the prone position. Lock the client's calf using reinforced thumbs, just distal to the knee joint, perhaps in the centre of the calf. Each time you lock the fibres in this stretch, direct your pressure towards the knee rather than perpendicularly. Never press directly into the popliteal space at the back of the knee. Whilst maintaining your lock, use your thigh to dorsiflex the client's ankle. Note that in this position, it is doubtful whether pressure applied by the therapist is deep enough to affect soleus. STR to soleus would be performed with your client in a side-lying position.

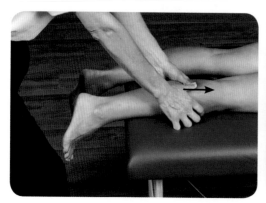 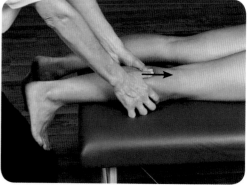

TIP Take care when using your thumbs. The calf muscle are strong and powerful. If you find that using your thumbs here to apply passive STR causes you discomfort, switch to a different method.

Another method of applying passive STR to the calf is to use your fists to apply the lock.

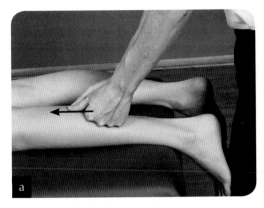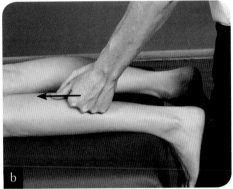

Applying a fist lock (a) and stretching the calf (b).

A slightly different method of using passive STR on the calf is to position your client prone, his or her knee flexed and his or her leg resting on your thigh. In this position you can glide your forearm along the length of the calf, using oil, as you dorsiflex the foot and ankle. This is an example of working distally to proximally. The client will sense more of a stretch just above the Achilles tendon and into the belly of the calf compared to when you glide closer to the knee. Another reason for the stretch to be felt more intensely is that with the knee flexed, gastrocnemius is relaxed, facilitating a stretch of the underlying soleus.

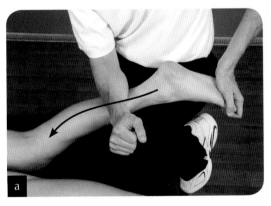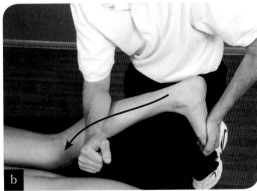

Applying a forearm lock to the calf (a) and gliding along the muscle (b).

Similarly, can you see how you could modify the use of fists so that instead of working your way from the knee to the ankle using static locks each time you dorsiflex the foot and ankle, you could begin close to the Achilles tendon and simply glide your fists up the length of the calf, with oil, as you passively dorsiflex-and-relax, and dorsiflex-and-relax the client's foot and ankle?

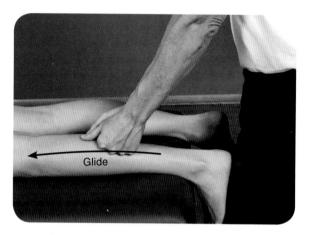

Using fists to apply gliding STR to the calf.

Hamstrings

With your client in the prone position, passively shorten the hamstring muscles by flexing the client's knee. Lock the muscle close to the origin at the ischium. Each time you lock the fibres in this stretch, direct your pressure towards the ischium rather than perpendicularly. Whilst maintaining your lock, gently stretch the muscle by extending the knee.

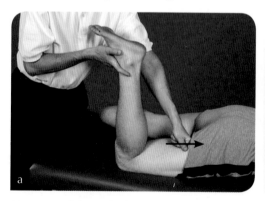 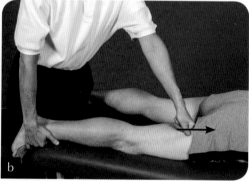

Using a soft fist to lock (a) and stretch (b) the hamstrings.

> **TIP** If you are working with a client with long legs, or who has a stature taller than yours, and it is difficult for you to apply locks close to the ischium or the upper part of the hamstring, then choose to focus only on the lower part of the muscle, or select a different method of STR, rather than strain your back in an attempt to lean across the massage couch to reach your client.

Gluteals

You can apply passive STR to the gluteal muscles using the elbow. Due to the shape of these muscles, it is not possible to work along the length of the fibres as you might when working on a longitudinal area of soft tissue such as the hamstrings or biceps brachii. In the case of the gluteal muscles you simply work over the area, changing the position of your lock until you and your client sense a stretch has occurred. To achieve the stretch, you will need to passively rotate the client's femur; an easy way to do so is simply to move the foot of the limb on which you are working towards or away from you.

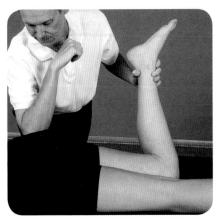 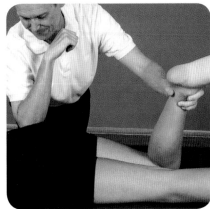

Rhomboids

There are two methods of applying STR to rhomboids. The first is with your client prone on a treatment couch, and the second is with your client seated. When treating the client in prone, position your client on the treatment couch so that he or she is able to flex at the shoulder. Whilst holding the client's arm to keep the rhomboids passively shortened, gently lock them, directing your pressure towards the spine. Maintain your lock and gently lower the arm into flexion so that the scapula protracts around the rib cage, stretching the rhomboids.

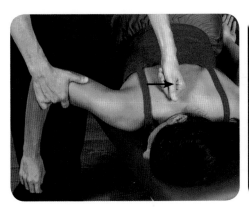 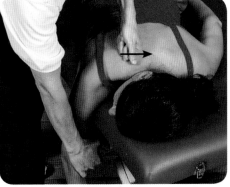

Alternatively, with your client comfortably seated, gently hold the arm to passively retract the scapula, which shortens the rhomboids. Take up the slack in the skin, directing your pressure towards the spine. Whilst maintaining your lock, take the arm into flexion, passively protracting the scapula.

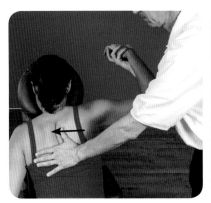 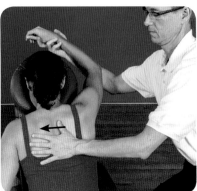

Using the thumb in this way requires little force, as the skin is fairly loose when the scapula is retracted in this position. However, if using your thumb to create the lock causes you discomfort, you should opt for a different method.

Triceps

Position your client in the prone position, and make sure he or she is able to flex the arm at the elbow. Take care not to squash the cubital fossa against the couch as you work from the shoulder to the elbow. Passively extend your client's elbow to shorten the muscle. Place your lock close to the origin, directing your pressure towards the shoulder. Whilst maintaining your lock, gently flex the elbow. In this example, the therapist has chosen to grip the triceps gently as the client is of slender frame and a firm grip or different lock is not needed in this instance. If you wanted to use your fist or thumb to apply the lock, pressure would need to be directed towards the armpit. When working with a client with long arms, you cannot apply STR all the way towards the distal end of the triceps muscle, because you may find that the client's arm is not supported on the couch.

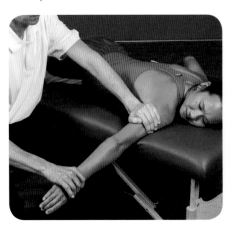 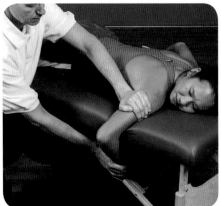

Shoulder Adductors

With your client prone and his or her elbow comfortably relaxed and flexed, it is possible to apply passive STR to the inferior portion of the shoulder without damaging structures of the armpit. This stretch requires you to press gently into the soft tissues, creating a lock with one hand, then using your other hand to gently traction the shoulder joint. Whilst retaining both the lock and traction, you then gently abduct your client's arm.

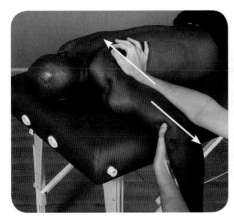 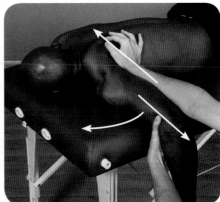

Biceps Brachii

With your client in supine and his or her elbow passively flexed, lock in gently to the biceps brachii, taking up slack in the skin as you direct pressure towards the armpit. Gently extend the elbow whilst maintaining your lock. In the example, the therapist is standing closer to the couch than normal so that you can see the position of the lock he has created with his left thumb. If he were to apply pressure in this position it would be slightly uncomfortable for his thumb. In practice, he would move away from the couch slightly, blocking the view of his hand, so that pressure was applied down the length of his forearm, wrist and thumb, with his joints in a 'stacked' position.

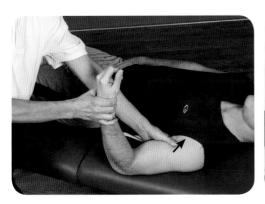 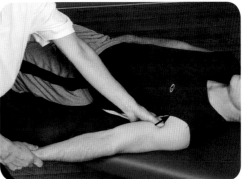

As when working on the calf muscle, you can modify STR so that, with oil, you glide along the biceps brachii muscle, working from the elbow to the shoulder. When working this way simply begin with a flexed elbow and as you glide your first, for example, along the muscle, gently flex–extend and flex–extend the client's elbow.

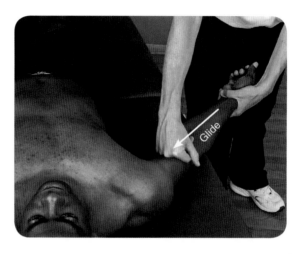

Wrist and Finger Extensors

To apply passive STR to the wrist and finger extensor muscles, gently extend your client's wrist, then lock into the bellies of the extensors on the lateral aspect of the forearm. Direct your pressure towards the elbow. Whilst maintaining your lock, gently flex the wrist.

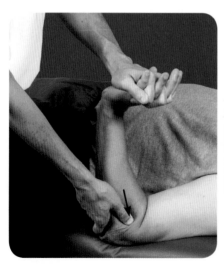
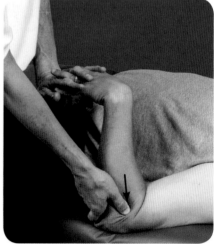

If you wanted to modify the technique to incorporate with massage when your client was in the prone position, simply position your client with the shoulder abducted, the forearm resting on the couch and the hand off the end of the couch. You can then glide from the wrist to the elbow whilst passively flexing-and-extending and flexing-and-extending the wrist.

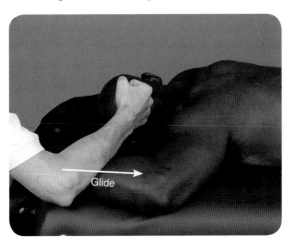

Wrist and Finger Flexors

Ask your client to flex the elbow. Gently lock into the common flexor origin. Gently extend the client's wrist whilst maintaining your lock.

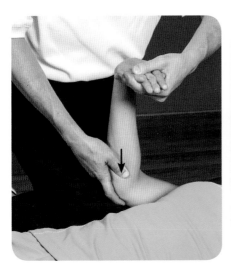
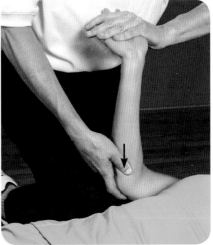

Pectorals

With your client in the supine position, take the arm into horizontal flexion and fix the tissues with a soft fist, directing your pressure towards the sternum rather than into the underlying ribs. Whilst maintaining your lock, gently take your client's arm from horizontal flexion into a more neutral position.

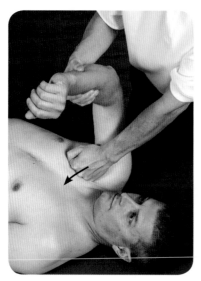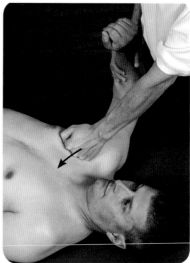

Notice that in the preceding photos, the therapist is choosing to use his left fist to lock the tissues, and with his right hand passively extends the client's shoulder. In the following photo, the therapist is working on a different client and has chosen to use his right fist to lock the tissues and his left to move the arm. In both cases the therapist is working on the client's right pectoral muscles. It does not matter which hand you use to lock tissues and which to move the arm. You may find that you have a preference or that you need to use different hands when working with different clients.

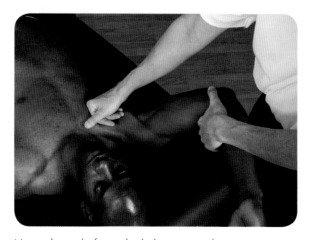

Using the right fist to lock the pectorals.

Safety Guidelines for Passive STR

Passive STR is safe and effective. However, it is useful to be aware of the following cautions before practising this technique.

- When applying STR to the calf with your client in the prone position, make sure there are no locking clips on your treatment couch that may injure the dorsal surface of your client's foot during dorsiflexion.

- When working with your client in prone to apply STR to the calf or hamstrings, avoid pressing into the popliteal space at the back of the knee.

- When working rhomboids in prone, be careful not to place your client's entire body to the side of the treatment couch. It is safer and more stable to have your client lie diagonally across the couch.

- Whilst working the biceps brachii, avoid putting pressure into the cubital fossa.

- Similarly, when working on triceps with your client prone, be careful not to squash the cubital fossa as you flex the elbow.

- When applying STR, protect your thumbs. If you find your client does not experience a sensation of stretch and needs a firmer lock, use an alternate lock. If you find that using a different lock places stress on your own body, consider using active-assisted STR, which often enables you to apply greater pressure and alter your stance to a safer working position.

- When integrating STR with oil massage, remember that it is much easier to provide a lock when working through a towel than when working through clothing or on dry skin. For this reason, apply your locks cautiously until you gain feedback from the client as to the appropriateness of your pressure.

- When using passive STR, always get feedback from your client and stop if the client reports pain.

- When applying passive STR, all the usual massage contraindications apply. For example, do not apply STR to areas with varicose veins, broken skin, recent injuries or decreased sensitivity.

- Passive STR to the shoulder adductors requires gentle traction of the shoulder joint so would be contraindicated in a client prone to shoulder subluxation.

When Is Passive STR Indicated?

Passive STR may be used directly through clothing all over the body as part of a general stretching routine, or it may be incorporated into a holistic massage treatment. It is useful when used briskly before exercise with the aim of increasing joint range of motion and overcoming cramps. It is used after exercise to help realign muscle fibres and overcome cramps. However, in both pre- and post-exercise settings, it should not be applied too deeply. It is also a useful tool for assessing muscle pliability.

Table 3.1 provides suggestions for when treatment for particular muscles can be useful.

Table 3.1 Situations in Which Passive STR Can Help

Muscle	Situation
Calf	<ul><li>To treat calf muscle cramps</li><li>For clients with tight calves</li><li>For clients engaged in physical activity involving the lower limbs, such as running, tennis or basketball</li><li>To treat clients who have been standing or walking for long periods</li><li>To increase range of motion at the ankle or knee</li><li>To treat clients who require increased ankle dorsiflexion (e.g., clients previously bedridden now required to stand)</li><li>To stretch out the calf muscles of clients who wear high-heeled footwear (which results in excessive plantar flexion and possible shortening of these muscles)</li></ul>
Hamstrings	<ul><li>For clients with tight hamstrings</li><li>For clients who sit for long periods, such as drivers or typists</li><li>For clients engaged in physical activity involving the lower limbs, such as running or basketball</li><li>To increase range of motion at the knee</li><li>For clients with excessive lumbar lordosis</li></ul>
Rhomboids	<ul><li>For clients engaged in physical activity involving the upper limbs, such as swimming, racquet sports or rowing</li></ul>
Triceps	<ul><li>For clients whose physical activities involve prolonged or repetitive extension of the elbow, such as in racquet sports</li><li>For massage therapists</li><li>For treatment after immobilization of the elbow or shoulder</li><li>To increase elbow flexion</li></ul>
Biceps brachii	<ul><li>For clients whose physical activities involve prolonged or repetitive elbow flexion, such as rowing, digging or carrying</li><li>For treatment after immobilization of the elbow or shoulder</li><li>To increase range of movement at the elbow, particularly elbow extension</li></ul>
Wrist and finger extensors and flexors	<ul><li>For musicians such as guitarists, pianists, flautists or trumpet players</li><li>In the treatment of lateral epicondylitis (extensors)</li><li>In the treatment of medial epicondylitis (flexors)</li><li>For clients who perform repeated or prolonged flexion, such as typists, drivers or people carrying heavy bags</li><li>For clients whose sport requires gripping, such as in rock climbing or rowing</li><li>For massage therapists</li><li>For treatment after immobilization of the wrist or elbow</li></ul>
Pectorals	<ul><li>For clients with kyphotic postures</li><li>For clients who sit for long periods of time, such as drivers or typists</li><li>For bodybuilders, who may develop excessively tight pectorals relative to posterior trunk muscles</li><li>For clients who use the pectoralis major as part of their job, hobby or sport, such as trumpet players, tennis players or golfers</li></ul>

Using Passive STR to Treat Trigger Points

When using passive STR to treat trigger points, you will need to use either your thumb or your elbow. If you are not familiar with treating trigger points, using your thumb will be easiest. Instead of working down the muscle, creating new locks, you remain in one position, your thumb (or elbow) over the trigger point. Use these steps as a guide:

1. Shorten the muscle you intend to work on.
2. Palpate the area to locate a trigger point, using feedback from the client to guide you.
3. Place your thumb gently over the point, and apply pressure. Get feedback from your client: pressure should feel slightly uncomfortable but not painful. Remember, pain causes muscles to tense and so is counterproductive to STR stretching.
4. Maintaining your lock, gently lengthen the muscle, stretching the fibres.
5. Release your lock, and soothe the area.
6. Feel for the trigger point again, and again get feedback from your client as you repeat the technique a total of four or five times.

How will you know if you have successfully treated a trigger point? First, the point should feel less firm to touch, and the client should report less discomfort (if any) when the point is pressed. Symptoms associated with the trigger may reduce, although in most cases it is likely to take more than one session for this reduction to occur. To elicit the same level of discomfort, you are likely to need to press deeper into the muscle. When triggers are first touched, very little pressure is needed to elicit discomfort. So it is a handy, rough guide as to how effective your passive STR has been in reducing a trigger point.

How to Become Proficient in the Use of Passive STR

As described in chapter 2, the three types of STR are passive, active-assisted and active. One way you could become proficient in the application of passive STR is to use table 3.2, making notes for yourself as you practise on each of the muscles, using various locks. Here are some ideas to help you get the most out of your practice sessions:

- Practise on each of the muscles, using the techniques shown, at least two times.
- Determine whether you prefer using your thumbs, fist or forearm to create a lock, and on which muscles they work best for you. It is unlikely that you will want to use your thumbs to apply STR to each of the muscles discussed in this chapter, for example, and more likely that you will develop a preference for using a particular lock when working on a particular muscle, using a variety of different locks in your overall practice.

■ You need to get feedback from the person on whom you are practising. Just because one person reports preferring to receive passive STR when you use your fist on their biceps brachii, for example, doesn't mean that all recipients will prefer this method of locking. Therefore, practising different locks can be advantageous in order to meet the preferences of different clients.

■ For each muscle you work on, experiment with changing from using your right hand to create the lock to using your left hand to create the lock.

■ Think about how your body feels as you practise. Are you comfortable? Raising or lowering your treatment couch can make a big difference to how comfortable you feel whilst working.

Quick Questions

1. What does it mean to say that a muscle is in a neutral position?
2. In passive STR, who performs the stretch—the client or the therapist?
3. Is a lock maintained whilst the muscle is being stretched?
4. Where is the client most likely to feel the stretch—at the proximal or the distal end of the muscle?
5. Why should you be cautious when first integrating passive STR with oil massage?

Table 3.2   Overview of Passive STR Applications

Calf			

Prone
Reinforced thumbs
	Prone
	Fists
		Prone
		Forearm to apply
		  gliding technique
			Prone
			Fists to apply gliding
			  technique

Hamstrings	Gluteals	Rhomboids	
Prone Fists	Prone Elbow	Prone Fists	Seated Thumb

Triceps	Shoulder adductors	Biceps	

Prone
Grip
	Prone
	Palm combined with
	  gentle shoulder traction
		Supine
		Thumb
			Supine
			Fist to apply gliding
			  technique

Wrist and finger extensors		Wrist and finger flexors	Pectorals
Supine Thumb	Prone Forearm to apply gliding technique	Supine Thumb	Supine Fist

Active-Assisted Soft Tissue Release

This chapter will help you understand how to perform active-assisted STR. Safety guidelines and a table (4.2) will help you decide when active-assisted STR may be indicated for your clients. Table 4.3 provides an overview of all of the application examples provided in this chapter; you can use it when practising on each muscle. Test whether you have understood the principles by answering the Quick Questions at the end of the chapter.

Introduction to Active-Assisted Soft Tissue Release

Unlike passive STR (where tissues are shortened and locked by the therapist) or active STR (where the client performs the technique), active-assisted STR combines the efforts of both client and therapist. It is useful for working with clients who find it difficult to relax during treatment and also for those who like to be engaged with their treatment. It also enables the practitioner to apply more pressure when locking tissues, as might occur when treating clients who do not feel the stretch of passive STR. Active-assisted STR enables the therapist to use both hands if necessary to apply a firmer lock, which is helpful when treating large, bulky muscles such as hamstrings and quadriceps. Ability to reinforce a lock also enables you to safeguard your wrists, fingers and thumbs.

Active-assisted STR is particularly useful as part of the rehabilitation process after joint immobilization. Not only does it facilitate an increased range of motion in the joint, it also contributes to improving strength in the associated muscles. This strengthening occurs because the client is actively engaged in using the muscle being treated or the opposing muscle. It is a valuable rehabilitation technique and may be a safer post-surgery application than passive STR, because clients are encouraged to work within their pain-free range. With permission from medical personnel, it may be used early in the rehabilitation process to help keep joints lubricated, and active movement may encourage a better alignment of collagen fibres than might otherwise occur if the joint were left immobile.

The biggest difference between active-assisted and passive STR is that in passive STR, the therapist is stretching a relaxed muscle. In active-assisted STR, the muscle being stretched might be contracting eccentrically as the client uses it to move the associated joint.

How to Perform Active-Assisted STR

To perform active-assisted STR, follow these steps:

1. *Identify the muscle to be stretched and the direction of the fibres.*

2. *Ensure the muscle is in a neutral or shortened position.* Neutral means that the muscle is neither shortened too much nor stretched; it is the position you need your client to hold when you lock the tissues.

3. *Explain the procedure to the client.* Demonstrate the movement you want your client to perform once you have locked the tissues. If, for example, you want to shorten the hamstrings, you could simply say, 'Please bend your knee', and most clients would understand this instruction. However, when treating fibularis (formerly known as peroneals) and wrist flexors and extensors, for example, you need to be much more specific and demonstrate the action you want the client to perform (see sidebar). Many clients would not understand the command to evert the foot (needed for treating fibularis muscles) and would need to be shown what to do when asked to flex or extend the wrist.

4. *In the neutral or contracted position, lock the muscle to fix the fibres.* Where possible, start proximally, nearest to the origin of the muscle.

5. *Whilst maintaining your lock, ask your client to move in such a way that he or she feels a stretch in the muscle.* How the client moves will vary depending on which muscle you are working. (See chapters 6 to 8 for photographs, tips and additional descriptions of the movements for each muscle.)

6. *Once the muscle has been stretched, release your lock.* Then, either let the muscle return to neutral or ask your client to contract the muscle again.

7. *Choose another point to fix the muscle.* Work proximally to distally until you reach the distal tendons of the muscle.

Take a look at table 4.1. It compares muscles that are normally treated by starting with them in the neutral position with muscles that are shortened prior to STR. Neutral positions are used when treating the calf, foot, upper fibres of the

Ankle and Wrist Movements Clients Need to Perform During Active-Assisted STR

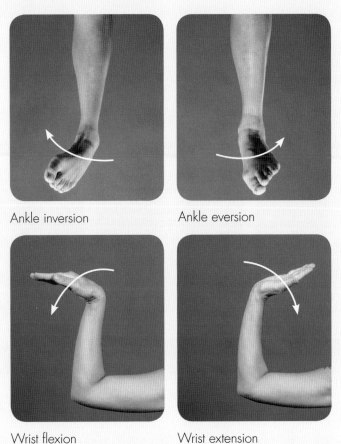

Ankle inversion   Ankle eversion

Wrist flexion   Wrist extension

trapezius, scalenes, levator scapulae, erector spinae, gluteal muscles and the ilio-tibial band (ITB). When a muscle needs to be shortened—as with the hamstrings, iliacus, tibialis anterior, peroneals, quadriceps, pectorals, biceps brachii, triceps and the wrist flexors and extensors—this shortening is performed by the client actively contracting the muscle in question.

The advantage of starting with a muscle in a shortened position is that it provides the possibility of the associated joint being moved through the entire joint range whereas when you begin with the muscle in a neutral position, there is less joint range to move through. Take a look at figure 4.1, which shows the ankle joint in these various positions: dorsiflexed (a), neutral (b) and plantarflexed (c).

Table 4.1   Comparing Start Positions

Neutral	Shortened
Calf	Hamstrings
Foot	Iliacus
Upper fibres of trapezius	Tibialis anterior
Scalenes	Fibularis (peroneals)
Levator scapulae	Quadriceps
Erector spinae	Pectorals
Gluteals	Biceps brachii
Iliotibial band (ITB)	Triceps
	Wrist flexors
	Wrist extensors

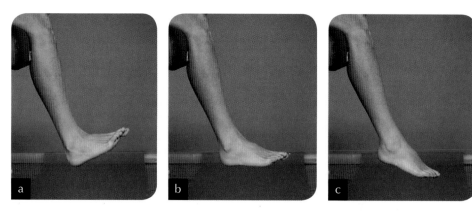

Figure 4.1   The ankle joint in dorsiflexed (*a*), neutral (*b*) and plantar flexed (*c*) positions.

Compare figure 4.2 with figure 4.3. Can you see how, if you begin with the ankle in plantar flexion it moves through a greater range (figure 4.2) than when you begin with it in neutral (figure 4.3)?

Another advantage of beginning with a muscle in a shortened position is that it is more effortful for a client to contract a muscle in order to take a joint through the entire range than it is for you to begin with a muscle in neutral, where no activation is required by the client at that time. This might be helpful where strengthening of that muscle is one of the treatment goals. Conversely, the constant repetition of starting with a muscle in a shortened position can be fatiguing for some clients. You can easily test this idea for yourself by contracting your tibialis muscle, fully dorsiflexing your foot and ankle as shown in figure 4.1*a*. Weaker than its plantar flexed counterpart, gastrocnemius, you only need to practise strong dorsiflexion three or four times to notice that the muscle starts to ache.

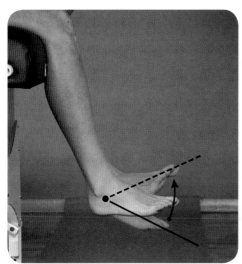 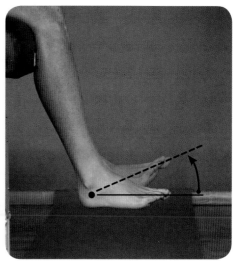

Figure 4.2 Moving through the entire ankle range from plantar flexion to dorsiflexion.

Figure 4.3 Moving through a partial ankle range, from neutral position to dorsiflexion.

Selecting Passive or Active-Assisted STR

You may be asking yourself, 'How do I know whether to begin with a muscle in a shortened position or a neutral position?' The answer is that you begin with some muscles in a neutral position because it would be difficult to either apply the lock or to take up slack in the skin if that same muscle were in a shortened position.

When treating clients, avoid swapping between passive STR and active STR initially. If you use both methods, you may find that clients get confused and forget whether they are supposed to be taking part in the stretch or relaxing and letting you move the associated joint. However, many clients soon learn what it is they are required to do for active-assisted STR, especially if they are receiving regular treatment from you. In subsequent treatments, you may find that you instinctively know which form of STR works best for which client; it is likely to vary depending on which muscle you are treating.

Remember that some clients never want to be actively engaged in their treatment, so active-assisted STR will never be appropriate, even in situations when you would view it as being beneficial. Some clients will always prefer the technique to be applied passively.

The Direction of Locks

As with passive STR, where possible you place your first lock at the proximal end of the muscle and work proximally to distally, as shown in figure 4.4.

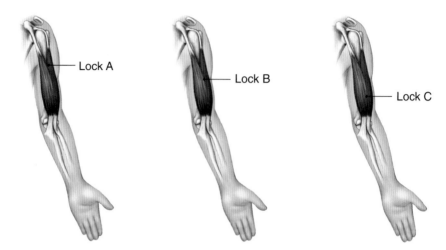

Figure 4.4   Direction in which locks are placed goes from lock A to lock B to lock C.

How to Focus the Stretch to One Area

This goal is achieved in exactly the same way as when using passive STR. Instead of using broad locks (figure 4.5) using a forearm, use your thumb or elbow to lock tissues successively in a smaller area (figure 4.6)

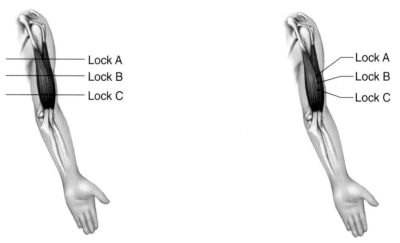

Figure 4.5   Applying broad, general locks.   **Figure 4.6**   Applying specific, localized locks.

The Direction of Pressure

When working on a limb, usually you press tissues away from you. In chapter 3 you learned that when applying passive STR it is necessary to counter the direction of drag that occurs when soft tissues lengthen. The same is true when applying active-assisted STR. For example, when working on levator scapulae and the upper fibres of trapezius it is necessary to apply gentle pressure downwards towards the scapula as you lock tissues (figure 4.7), and when working on the erector spinae to counter the drag in tissues caused by neck flexion, press gently downwards once you have locked the skin (figure 4.8).

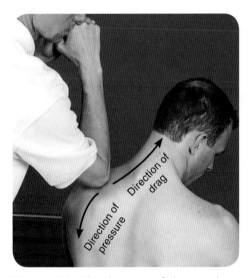

Figure 4.7   The direction of drag and direction of counterpressure when applying STR to levator scapulae.

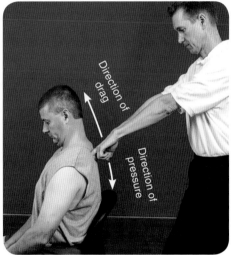

Figure 4.8   The direction of drag and direction of counterpressure when applying STR to erector spinae.

In the section titled Key Holds, Moves and Stances for Active-Assisted STR later in this chapter, arrows have been added to the photographs indicating the direction of pressure.

Taking Up Slack in the Skin

Compare figure 4.9 with the corresponding photograph for passive STR from chapter 3. Can you see how, in both cases, the therapist has gently taken up some slack in the skin as the tissues have been locked, making it a more effective stretch?

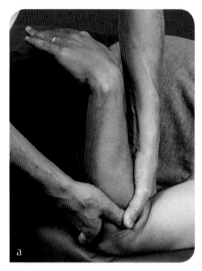 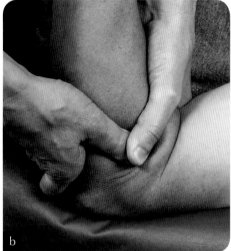

Figure 4.9 Taking up slack in the skin.

Incorporating Active-Assisted STR With Oil Massage

The easiest way to incorporate active-assisted STR with an oil massage is to keep a facecloth or very small towel to hand and, at the time when you are ready to apply STR, cover the area with the facecloth and apply your locks through it, adjusting it if necessary as you move along the muscle. The facecloth helps provide grip to the tissues. Without a cloth, tissues cannot be locked if a massage medium has been applied. Once you have finished applying STR, remove the cloth and continue to massage the area.

An alternative is to use gliding STR. Figures 4.10 through 4.12 illustrate three examples of when gliding might be used with active-assisted STR. Active-assisted STR gliding requires the client to dorsiflex and plantar flex repeatedly as you glide along the tibialis anterior muscle from ankle to knee.

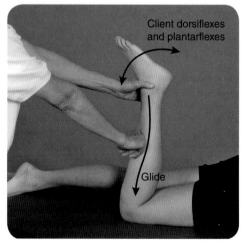

Figure 4.10 Using gliding STR on tibialis anterior.

Similarly, to work on the medial aspect of the calf when the client is in a side-lying position, glide gently from ankle to knee as the client dorsiflexes and plantar flexes. In the photograph the therapist has chosen to keep the client's foot and ankle on the couch, but other therapists encounter less resistance if either the foot is or foot and ankle are off the couch, providing the leg itself is supported.

In this third example, the therapist is using gliding active-assisted STR whilst running a cupped fist along the ITB from knee to hip as the client repeatedly flexes and extends the knee. As you can see, when gliding is used on the ITB the client needs to be in a comfortable side-lying position, the knee able to flex and extend, taking the leg off and onto the couch.

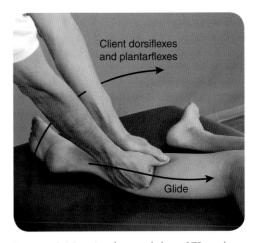

Figure 4.11 Applying gliding STR to the medial side of the calf.

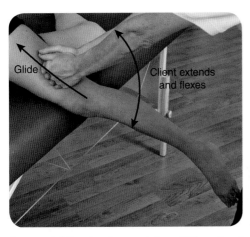
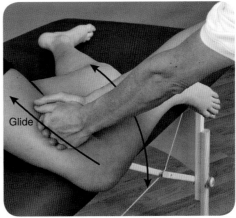

Figure 4.12 Applying gliding STR to the iliotibial band (ITB).

Key Holds, Moves and Stances for Active-Assisted STR

Illustrated here are 16 areas of the body that lend themselves to active-assisted STR: the calf, foot, hamstrings, iliacus, tibialis anterior, fibularis (peroneals), gluteals, quadriceps and ITB of the lower limbs; the upper trapezius, scalenes, levator scapulae, erector spinae and pectorals of the trunk; the wrist and finger extensors and flexors; and infraspinatus, biceps brachii and triceps. You can find detailed instructions for these stretches in chapters 6 through 8, where you can compare them to the passive and active techniques.

Calf

Lock the calf muscle just inferior to the knee joint, taking care not to press into the popliteal space at the back of the knee. Use your elbow, thumbs or forearm. Whilst maintaining your lock, ask your client to pull up his or her toes, thus dorsiflexing the foot and ankle. Next, remove your lock and move to a new position.

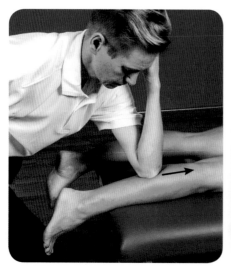 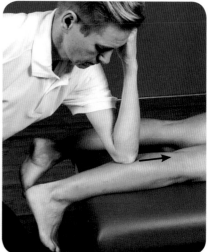

TIP On bulky calves it can be tricky to lock the tissues so use your other hand to cup your elbow for stability.

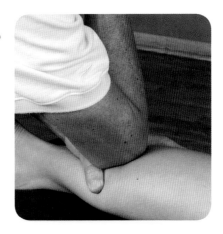

If you wish to create a specific lock but are finding it difficult to use your elbow, try locking the tissues using your thumbs.

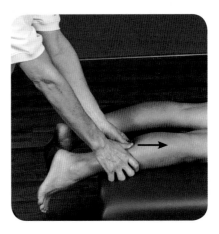

Alternatively, use your forearm if you wish to create a broad lock.

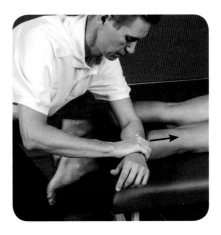

An adaptation of active-assisted STR is to grip the calf muscle as your client dorsiflexes and plantar flexes the foot and ankle.

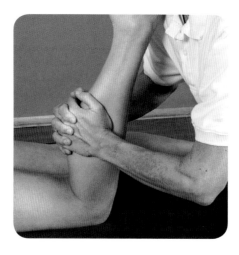

Foot

Position your client with his or her feet off the couch as shown; with the ankle in a neutral position, apply a gentle lock using a massage tool. Ask your client to pull up the toes, thus dorsiflexing the ankle and extending the toes. Work over the sole of each foot for a few minutes only.

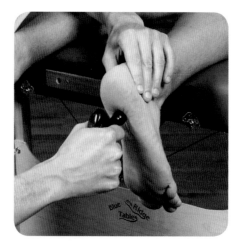

TIP If your client is ticklish when you work on the foot this way, simply work through a towel. You will need to apply a little massage medium first so that the fronds of the towel have something to grip. It also means you can apply less pressure, which can be helpful when working with clients with sensitive feet.

When working with a client in the supine position, the foot does not need to be off the couch because the client can obviously dorsiflex the ankle and extend the toes comfortably without the couch being in the way.

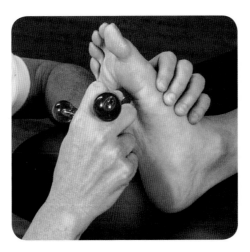

Hamstrings

Whilst your client is in a prone position, ask him or her to flex the knee. Lock the hamstrings close to the ischium. Direct your pressure towards the buttock to take up some of the slack in soft tissues before the stretch. Whilst maintaining your lock, ask your client to lower the leg back to the couch. Release your lock, and ask the client to flex the knee again.

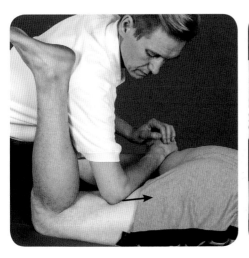
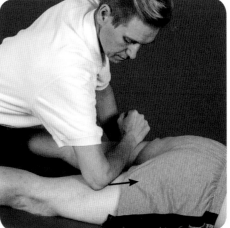

Practicing active-assisted STR is a good opportunity to experiment with swapping between using your right and left forearm. Notice that in the preceding photographs the therapist has chosen to apply STR to a client's right hamstring using the therapist's right forearm. Compare this sequence to the following photograph showing the therapist using the left forearm on the client's right hamstrings.

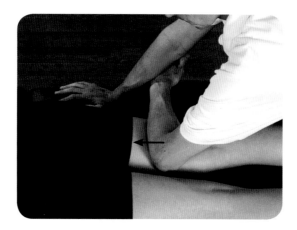

Using your elbow on the hamstrings creates a much more specific lock but is necessary when working with some clients who do not feel the stretch when you use other types of locks.

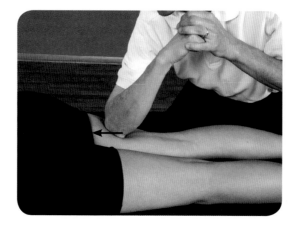

Iliacus

With your client positioned side lying with hip flexed, lock into the iliacus (on the anterior surface of the ilium). If you are not sure where to locate the muscle, identify the iliac crest and then slide your fingers over it, into the region of the iliac fossa. Whilst maintaining your lock, ask your client to straighten his leg and extend his hip. This application is more invasive than in all of the other examples in this book, so be certain that your client understands where you need to place the lock and has given consent to so.

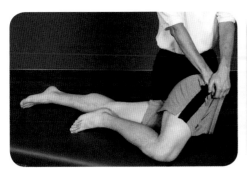 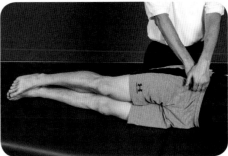

TIP When applying the lock to the iliacus, it is necessary to pull your fingertips towards you; in so doing, this action can rock the client backwards. Placing a cushion between your client and yourself helps provide stability and can help make clients feel more comfortable.

Tibialis Anterior

Whilst your client's ankle is in dorsiflexion, lock the tibialis anterior muscle using, for example, your elbow. Maintain your lock, and ask your client to point her toes. Then release your lock and choose a new position, slightly more distal, for your second lock. In the photo example, the therapist has chosen to apply STR with the client in a side-lying position, the leg supported on a bolster. You may prefer to use a bolster but find it best if the client's ankle is supported but her foot is not, thus facilitating dorsiflexion and plantar flexion.

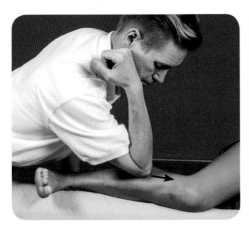 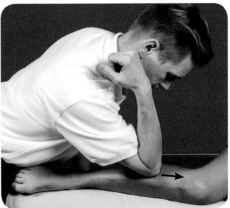

TIP When working on the tibialis anterior with your client in the side-lying position, take care at the proximal end of the muscle that you do not stray over to the head of the fibula, around which the common fibular nerve runs.

As an alternative, try using gliding STR.

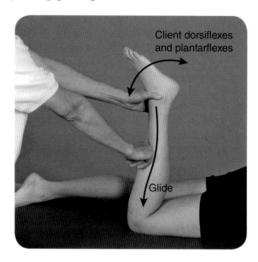

Fibularis (Peroneals)

With your client positioned in side lying, ask him or her to evert the foot. Lock the muscle, which is now in a shortened position. Whilst maintaining your lock, ask the client to invert the foot. Work in a single line down the muscle, from proximal to distal, so that the client feels the stretch and it remains comfortable. As when working on the tibialis anterior muscle with your client in the side-lying position, take care not to press into the area close to the head of the fibula as the common fibular nerve is located here.

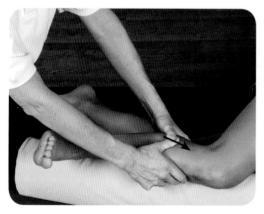 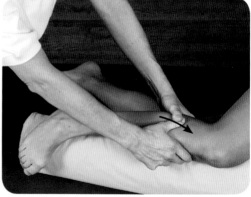

TIP With your client in the side-lying position, place his or her leg on a bolster to make it easier to invert the foot and ankle, which would otherwise be restricted by the couch.

Gluteals

With your client in the side-lying position, hip in neutral, use your forearm close to the elbow to lock the gluteals, directing your pressure towards the sacrum. Whilst maintaining your lock, ask your client to flex the hip. Repeat this action for a few minutes, working on the area that feels most beneficial for the client.

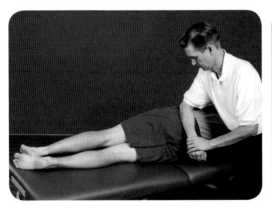
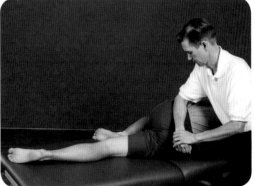

Quadriceps

With your client sitting, ask him or her to straighten the leg, which extends the knee. Once the muscle is actively shortened in this way, lock the quadriceps, taking up slack in soft tissues by easing them towards the hip. Whilst maintaining your lock, ask your client to flex the knee. Once the knee is flexed, release your lock and repeat, placing a new lock slightly more distal to the first. Work your way down the quadriceps from hip to knee. Notice that in the photograph the therapist has positioned the client so that not all of the thigh is supported on the couch. This positioning facilitates knee flexion but means that the therapist will not be able to apply locks close to the knee itself, at the distal end of the quadriceps muscles, as there will be no support from the couch. If you want to work on the distal end of the quadriceps, you will need to position your client so that the whole thigh is supported. However, you will need to compromise a little, as you client will only be able to flex the knee to around 90 degrees.

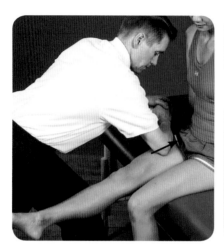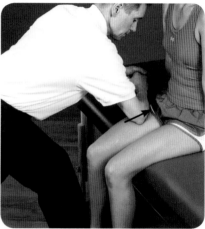

TIP To access the lateral side of the thigh, ask your client to lean away from you, transferring his or her weight onto the opposite buttock. The advantage to this position is that the lateral aspect of the thigh is then uppermost, but the disadvantage is that it can be tricky to find a suitable position in which to stand to avoid the client's foot touching you when flexing and extending the knee.

Iliotibial Band (ITB)

Position your client comfortably in a side-lying position. Ask him or her to straighten the leg, extending the knee. Starting just above the knee, lock the tissues, taking up slack where there is some by pressing tissues towards the hip. Retaining your lock, ask your client to bend the leg, flexing the knee. Repeat, using a series of locks as you work from the knee to the hip.

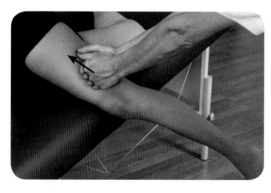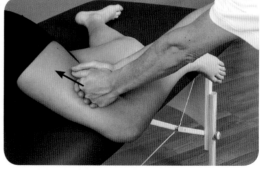

TIP Some clients find it much more comfortable if a sponge or small towel is placed between the knee and the couch of the leg on which they are resting.

CLIENT TALK

A recreational runner came for treatment because he felt that the lateral side of his left thigh was tight and pulling on his knee. He had tried using a foam roller but found this method extremely painful, and had difficulty getting into the correct position on the floor in order to rest on the roller. Although the client was advised to consider myofascial release as an effective treatment for this part of the thigh, his impression was that he required 'deep work'. The area was warmed thoroughly with massage and then active-assisted STR applied through a towel, using a combination of fists and palms. The client enjoyed this method, as he felt a deep stretch sensation, which he believed would be beneficial at alleviating his symptoms.

Upper Trapezius

With your client sitting, lock the upper fibres of the trapezius. Whilst maintaining your lock, ask your client to flex his or her neck laterally until he or she feels a comfortable stretch. Repeat the action three times, then repeat on the opposite side of the body. Notice how your lock gets dragged towards the ear slightly as your client laterally flexes the neck. To counter this movement, you need to direct your pressure gently away from the ear, toward the top of the shoulder, without pressing into the acromion, which would be uncomfortable for the client.

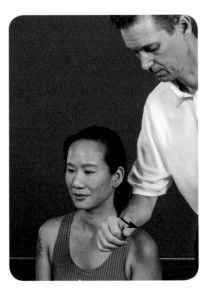 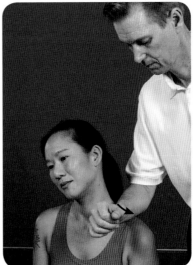

Another option is to use your thumbs, a massage tool or a tennis ball to lock into the upper fibres of the trapezius whilst your client is in the supine position. Once locked, ask your client to laterally flex the head and neck. For example, when locking the right trapezius you might ask the client to take the left ear to the left shoulder.

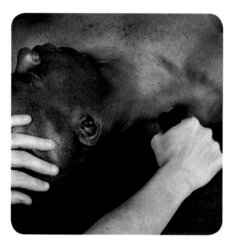 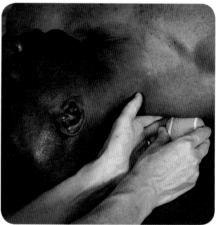

Scalenes

With your client sitting, gently lock the scalenes using your fingers. Ask your client to rotate his or her head away from you until he or she feels a comfortable stretch in the tissues. Perform the action three times on both the left and right sides. Notice how your fingers are drawn away from the clavicle as your client turns the head away from you. Counter this movement with very gentle pressure, taking care not to press too deeply.

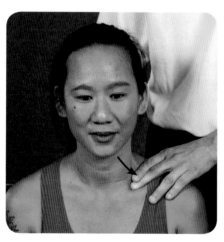 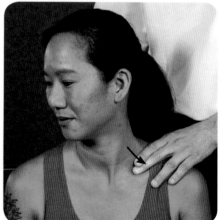

This technique is also effective when treating a client in the supine position.

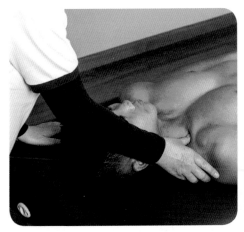 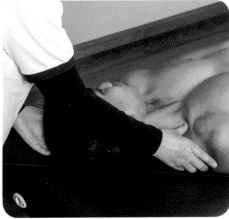

Levator Scapulae

Locate and lock the levator scapulae. Whilst maintaining your lock, ask your client to rotate the head to about 45 degrees and then lower the chin to look to the floor. Ask your client to repeat this stretch three times; then use the same stretch on the opposite side of the body. Notice how your elbow is drawn up towards the head as the client stretches. Counter this movement with gentle pressure in the opposite direction, towards the top of the scapula.

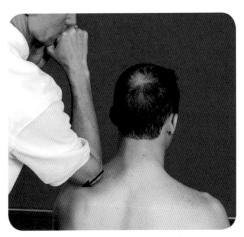 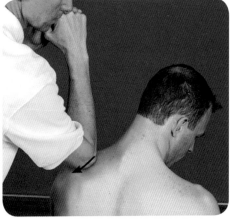

Erector Spinae (Spinalis)

With your client sitting, lock the tissues just below the neck. Whilst maintaining your lock, ask your client to flex the neck. Release and repeat, placing your lock slightly superior to the first one. To counter the drag of soft tissues into the neck, direct your lock into the tissues and to the floor at the same time. One of the challenges of applying active-assisted STR to erector spinae with a client seated is that there is a tendency to push the client forwards as you press into the tissues in an attempt to create a lock. One way to counter this movement is to have the client straddle the chair, with a pillow between his or her chest and the back of the chair.

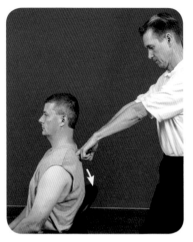 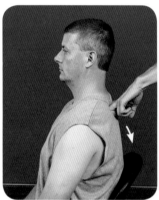 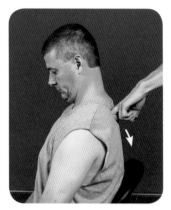

Pectorals

Ask your client to take his or her arm across the body, actively shortening pectoralis major. Using soft fists, lock the muscle, directing your pressure towards the sternum. Whilst maintaining your lock, ask your client to move the arm so that he or she feels a stretch in the pectorals.

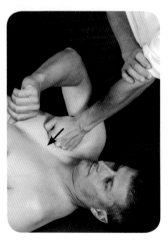 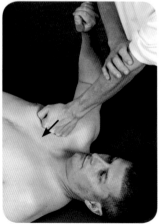

Wrist and Finger Extensors

Locate the bellies of the wrist and finger extensors by asking your client to extend the wrist. Lock the tissues, taking up slack in the skin by pressing gently towards the elbow. Whilst maintaining your lock, ask your client to flex the wrist. Repeat over the lateral aspect of the elbow where the muscle bellies are located.

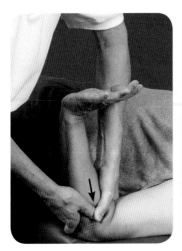 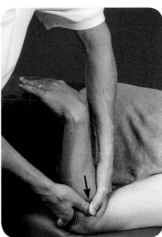

An effective way to apply active-assisted STR to the wrist extensors is with your client seated, his or her arm resting on the massage couch, the wrist able to flex freely over the end of the couch.

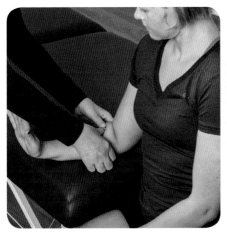 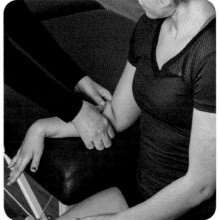

Notice how you could modify active-assisted STR to the wrist extensors by turning it into a gliding technique. With your client prone, his or her hand off the massage couch, begin at the wrist and using a massage medium, glide gently towards the elbow as your client flexes and extends the wrist.

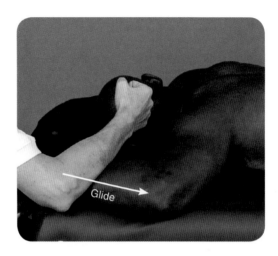

Wrist and Finger Flexors

Identify the muscles by asking the client to flex his or her wrist. Lock the tissues over the muscle bellies, directing your pressure gently towards the elbow. Whilst maintaining your lock, ask your client to extend the wrist. Repeat this lock, stretch, lock, stretch sequence over the muscle bellies.

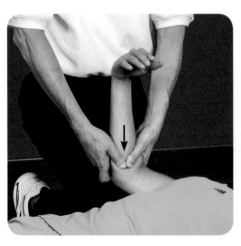
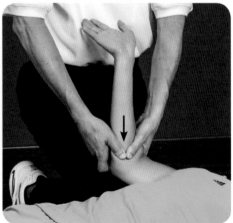

Infraspinatus

Active-assisted STR to infraspinatus is performed with your client in the prone position. It is important that you ask your client to rest with the arms by the sides, the palms touching the couch, at the start. In this position the infraspinatus is contracted. Use gentle pressure to apply a lock and, whilst maintaining the lock, ask your client to change the position of the arms by turning the hands so that the back of the hands are against the couch. There is no need to take up slack in the skin when applying a lock to this muscle.

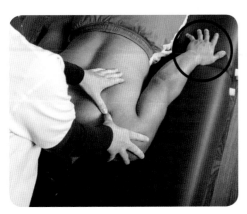 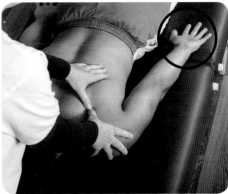

TIP There is a trigger point in the middle of the infraspinatus muscle that, in most people, feels tender when pressed. Using active-assisted STR on this very trigger point is useful in reducing tension in the shoulder.

Biceps Brachii

With your client in the supine position, ask him or her to flex the elbow. Then create a lock using either the back of your fingers, a soft knuckle or your thumb, taking up slack in the tissues as you press gently towards the shoulder. Maintaining your lock, ask your client to slowly extend the elbow.

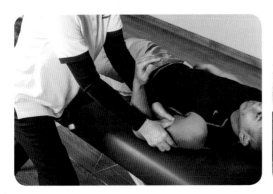 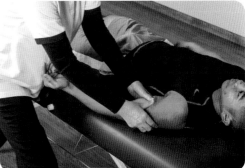

Triceps

You can use active-assisted STR to stretch the triceps in this manner: Gently abduct your client's arm whilst he or she is in the prone position, then ask him or her to extend the elbow. Lock the tissues gently at the proximal end of the muscle, taking up slack towards the shoulder. Maintaining this position, ask your client to flex his or her elbow. As with passive STR to triceps in this position, it is not always possible to stretch the distal end of the muscle when working with a client with long arms; when abducted, this part of the arm is not supported by the couch and you therefore have no resistance to the pressure of your lock.

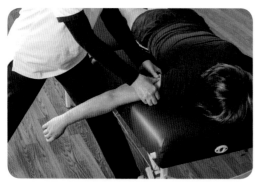 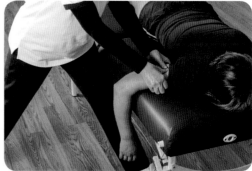

Safety Guidelines for Active-Assisted STR

The following guidelines will help keep active-assisted STR safe for you and your clients:

- Your usual massage contraindications apply. For example, do not apply active-assisted STR to the calf if your client has varicose veins.

- When treating the calf and hamstring muscles, avoid pressing into the popliteal space behind the knee.

- When working, be aware of your posture and guard your back. For example, avoid unsupported spinal flexion when treating the calf.

- When working with a client with an injury to the tibialis anterior, avoid applying active-assisted STR to the calf. In this case, constant dorsiflexion will fatigue the tibialis anterior. An exception may be when a client has a dropped foot due to weakness in the tibialis anterior; in this case, active-assisted STR to the calf may actually be beneficial as part of a programme to increase strength in the ankle dorsiflexors.

- When working along the tibia and fibula, ensure that the client's knee is fully supported if he or she is in side lying position. If you are applying your elbows to access these strap-like muscles, work cautiously to avoid bruising the tissues against the underlying bones. Take care not to press onto or close by the head of the fibula where the common fibular nerve runs.

■   When stretching the quadriceps of clients with anterior knee pain, recognize that you may not be able to work to as distal a point as usual. This limitation is because the closer to the knee you place your lock, the greater the stretch and the greater the pressure on the patella. Whilst it may be beneficial in the long term in overcoming patellofemoral pain due to tight quadriceps, it could be painful during the stretch itself.

■   When working the scalenes, take care not to press too deeply. Be sure to get feedback from the client.

■   Avoid using STR on the feet when a client has diabetes, unless you are certain they have full sensation in their feet and can feed back to you any discomfort.

■   Avoid using STR to levator scapulae or trapezius in the seated position with clients with low back problems; pressure through the body this way can aggravate symptoms.

When Is Active-Assisted STR Indicated?

Overall, active-assisted STR is useful in these situations:

■   When working with clients who find it difficult to relax during treatment

■   When treating clients who like to be engaged with their treatment

■   When it is necessary to apply more pressure to lock tissues

■   When treating clients who do not feel the stretch of passive STR

■   When treating large, bulky muscles such as hamstrings and quadriceps

■   When it is essential for you to safeguard your wrists, fingers and thumbs

■   When muscle strengthening is required, perhaps after immobilization of a joint

Table 4.2 provides suggestions for when active-assisted treatment to particular muscles may be useful.

Using Active-Assisted STR to Treat Trigger Points

When using active-assisted STR to treat trigger points, instead of working down the muscle, creating new locks, remain in one position, using your thumb over the trigger point as your client moves the joint in order to stretch the muscle you are working on. Because you do not need to move any part of the client's body, it is tempting to use both hands to apply pressure to a point, but it is unnecessary. Only light pressure is required. Use these steps as a guide:

1. Shorten the muscle you intend to work on.

2. Palpate the area to locate a trigger point, using feedback from the client to guide you.

Table 4.2　Situations in Which Active-Assisted STR Can Help

Muscle	Situation
Calf	<ul><li>For clients with tight calves</li><li>For clients engaged in physical activity involving the lower limbs, such as running, tennis or basketball</li><li>To treat clients who have been standing or walking for long periods</li><li>To increase range of motion at the ankle or knee</li><li>To treat clients who require increased ankle dorsiflexion (e.g., clients previously bedridden now required to stand)</li><li>To stretch out the calf muscles of clients who wear high-heeled footwear (which results in excessive plantar flexion and possible shortening of these muscles)</li><li>For use as part of a programme to help strengthen the tibialis anterior</li></ul>
Foot	<ul><li>For clients with plantar fasciitis</li><li>For clients with Achilles tendon problems</li></ul>
Hamstrings	<ul><li>For clients with tight hamstrings</li><li>For clients who sit for long periods, such as drivers or typists</li><li>For clients engaged in physical activity involving the lower limbs, such as cycling, running or basketball</li><li>To increase range of motion at the knee</li><li>For clients with excessive lumbar lordosis</li><li>With medical permission, after knee surgery or immobilization of the knee</li></ul>
Iliacus	<ul><li>For clients with tight hip flexors</li><li>For clients engaged in physical activity that requires repetitive or prolonged hip flexion, such as running, rowing, cycling or jockeying</li><li>For clients who sit for long periods, such as drivers</li><li>To increase hip extension</li><li>For clients engaged in riding motorcycles for long periods</li></ul>
Tibialis anterior	<ul><li>For clients with tight tibialis anterior muscles</li><li>For clients engaged in sporting activities that require repeated or prolonged dorsiflexion, such as running or tennis</li><li>After walking uphill for long periods</li><li>After standing for long periods</li><li>To help increase plantar flexion, should that be required, after ankle joint immobilization</li></ul>
Peroneals	<ul><li>For clients with tight peroneals, often those with flat feet</li><li>To help increase inversion after immobilization of the ankle joint</li><li>For clients engaged in physical activity that uses the leg muscles</li><li>For clients who are prone to repetitive eversion of the ankle, such as horse riders</li></ul>
Gluteals	<ul><li>For clients engaged in physical activity that requires repetitive or prolonged hip extension or abduction, such as running, jumping or ice skating</li></ul>

(continued)

Muscle	Situation
Quadriceps	■ For clients with tight quadriceps ■ For clients engaged in physical activity involving the lower limbs, such as cycling, running or jumping ■ To increase range of motion at the knee ■ To increase knee flexion
Upper trapezius, scalenes, levator scapulae, erector spinae (spinalis)	■ For clients with tight neck muscles ■ For clients who spend long periods sitting, such as writers, drivers or typists ■ For singers ■ To increase range of motion in the neck ■ For treatment after immobilization of the neck ■ During seated chair massage routines by therapists working in this capacity ■ For clients who suffer headaches induced by increased muscle tension ■ For clients needing treatment after immobilization of the scapula or as part of the rehabilitation process after injury to the shoulder, especially for the upper trapezius and levator scapulae ■ For anyone who performs repetitive or prolonged shoulder activities, especially those involving overarm movements, such as tennis, swimming or overarm bowling ■ For clients who hold static postures for prolonged periods, such as painters, artists or models
Pectorals	■ For clients with tight pectorals ■ For clients with kyphotic postures ■ To increase horizontal extension at the shoulder ■ For treatment after immobilization of the shoulder joint (when the client has been in a sling, for example) ■ For clients who perform repeated or prolonged movements of the shoulder, especially those activities requiring adduction, forward flexion and horizontal flexion of the shoulder, such as rock climbing, racquet sports or swimming ■ For clients who maintain prolonged forward flexion at the shoulder, such as cyclists or drivers
Wrist and finger extensors and flexors	■ For musicians whose performance requires repeated finger movements, such as guitarists, pianists, flautists or trumpet players ■ In the treatment of lateral epicondylitis (extensors) ■ In the treatment of medial epicondylitis (flexors) ■ For clients who perform repeated or prolonged flexion, such as typists, drivers or people who carry heavy bags ■ For clients whose sport requires gripping, such as rock climbing or rowing ■ For massage therapists ■ For treatment after immobilization of the wrist or elbow

3. Place your thumb gently over the point, and apply pressure. Get feedback from your client: pressure should feel slightly uncomfortable but not painful. Remember, pain causes muscles to tense and so is counterproductive to STR stretching.

4. Maintaining your lock, gently lengthen the muscle, stretching the fibres.

5. Release your lock, and soothe the area.

6. Feel for the trigger point again, and again get feedback from your client as you repeat the technique a total of four or five times.

As the trigger point dissipates, it will feel less firm to touch; the client should report less discomfort (if any) when the point is pressed. It usually takes more than one treatment session for all symptoms associated with the trigger to resolve.

How to Become Proficient in the Use of Active-Assisted STR

Use table 4.3 as you practise active-assisted STR on each of the muscles shown in this chapter, experimenting with different locks. To get the most out of your practice sessions you might wish to try the following:

- Practise changing your posture by raising or lowering your treatment couch.
- Alternate between using your right and left hands to create the lock. On which muscles do you need to reinforce the lock and use both hands?
- Practise with using gliding STR.
- Ask your client which locks he or she prefers the feel of and which provide the strongest or most comfortable stretch. Do any locks feel uncomfortable or not seem to work for either you or your client?
- Practise at least two times on each of the muscles.

Quick Questions

1. Who performs the stretch in active-assisted STR—the client, the therapist or both?
2. For which sort of client might active-assisted STR be useful?
3. Why is this form of STR useful for rehabilitation after joint immobilization?
4. What is the biggest difference between passive and active-assisted STR?
5. Why should you avoid swapping between passive and active-assisted STR when working with a client for the first time?

Table 4.3   Overview of Active-Assisted STR Applications

Calf

Prone Elbow	Prone Forearm	Prone Double thumbs	Prone Squeeze
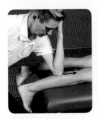	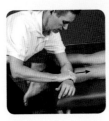	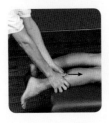	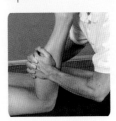

Foot | | Hamstrings

Prone Tool	Supine Tool	Prone Forearm	Prone Elbow
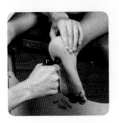	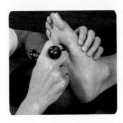	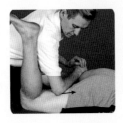	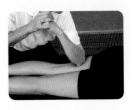

Iliacus | Tibialis anterior | | Fibularis

Side lying Fingers	Side lying Elbow	Prone Fist, gliding	Side lying Thumbs
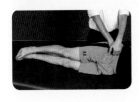	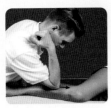	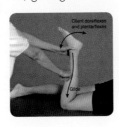	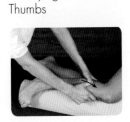

(continued)

Gluteals	Quadriceps	Scalenes	
Side lying Forearm/elbow	Seated Forearm	Seated Fingers	Supine Fingers

Iliotibial band (ITB)	Upper trapezius		
Side lying Fists	Seated Forearm	Supine Tool	Supine Tennis ball

Levator scapulae	Erector spinae	Pectorals	Infraspinatus
Seated Elbow	Seated Knuckles	Supine Soft fist	Prone Fingers

(continued)

Wrist extensors			Wrist flexors
Supine Thumbs	Seated Thumbs	Prone Forearm to apply gliding technique	Supine Thumbs

Biceps brachii	Triceps	
Supine Soft fist	Prone Thumbs	

Active Soft Tissue Release

Passive and active-assisted STR are techniques used when treating clients. In this chapter, you will discover how to perform active STR, a technique you might use on yourself or teach to your clients to use as part of a home care programme. Included are brief descriptions of the key holds, moves and stances used for treating 13 muscles, with accompanying photographs, along with safety guidelines and a table (5.1) illustrating when active STR may be indicated. As with the previous two chapters, this chapter provides an overview table (5.2) too. Answering the Quick Questions at the end of the chapter will help test your understanding of how active STR is applied.

Introduction to Active Soft Tissue Release

It is possible to perform active soft tissue release on many of the muscles in the body. To do so, you apply a lock to yourself and perform the stretch yourself, with no assistance from a therapist. Unlike passive soft tissue release, the muscle involved will be actively rather than passively shortened. In other words, you will lock into a contracted rather than a relaxed muscle. Nevertheless, the technique seems to be effective at releasing tension in the muscle and is useful as a quick fix when a therapist is unavailable. Active STR is invaluable as a method for treating trigger points.

How to Perform Active STR

To perform active STR, follow these steps:

1. *Identify the muscle to be stretched and the direction of the fibres.*
2. *Shorten the muscle.* In other words, concentrically contract it; how you contract it will depend on which muscle you are working. To contract your hamstrings, for example, flex your knee; to contract your triceps, extend your elbow. In some cases you do not need to contract the muscle in order to take a joint through its full range. In fact, doing so can make STR impossible. For example, if you contracted biceps to fully flex your elbow, you would not be able to lock the muscle because you would have no space to apply a lock.
3. *With the muscle gently shortened, lock the fibres.* Start proximally, nearest the origin of the muscle.
4. *Once the fibres are locked, actively lengthen the muscle.* Maintain your lock throughout the movement.
5. *Once the muscle is lengthened, remove your lock.*
6. *Shorten the muscle again.*
7. *Choose a new place to lock, slightly more distal to your first position.* Repeat the action.

Stop when you reach the distal tendons of the muscle. If you have performed STR correctly, you should feel the stretch increase as you work from proximal to distal on the muscle.

TIP To be really good at performing STR, you need to know your muscles and the actions they bring about. For reference, keep an anatomy text close at hand whilst working through this book and practising STR.

The Direction of Locks

When locking a muscle, the intensity of the subsequent stretch increases as you work from the proximal end of the muscle to the distal end. In figure 5.1, lock C produces a stretch of greater intensity than lock A because there is less soft tissue to stretch when locking the distal end of the muscle.

However, depending on the shape of the muscle and how you lock the tissues, it may not be possible to follow this guideline. For example, in figure 5.2 the subject has a large, bulky biceps muscle. Using a gripping lock, it is not possible to work from the proximal end to the distal end. Biceps brachii is a good example of where active STR may not be as effective as passive or active-assisted STR.

How to Focus the Stretch to One Area

Placing locks close together (figure 5.4) focuses a stretch to one area of tissue more accurately than when locks are placed farther apart (figure 5.3). In many cases,

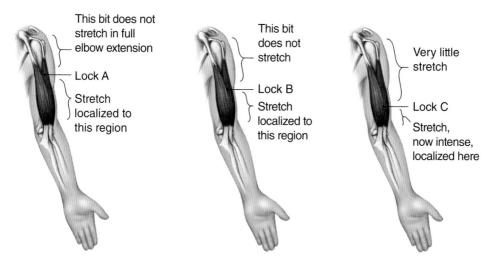

Figure 5.1   Locks placed proximally to distally increases the intensity of a stretch.

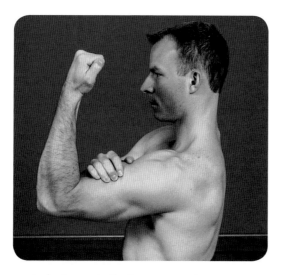

Figure 5.2   Using a grip lock to a bulky biceps muscle.

active STR works best when a tennis ball is used to create the lock. Be careful to avoid overworking any one area. The risk of overworking an area is slightly greater when using active STR compared to passive or active-assisted STR because when applying passive or active-assisted STR, these methods may already be incorporated into a massage routine, during which muscles are soothed following the application of locks. If prescribing active STR as a useful stretching method for your clients, ask them to self-massage the area wherever possible if they have localized a stretch to one particular muscle.

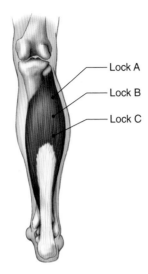

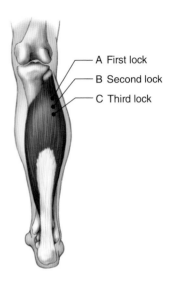

Figure 5.3 Specific locks spread across the length of the muscle.

Figure 5.4 Specific locks placed close together.

The Direction of Pressure

Usually when applying STR, pressure is directed towards the proximal end of the muscle. For example, when treating the wrist extensors (figure 5.5a) or flexors (figure 5.5b), you can use the thumb to direct pressure towards the elbow.

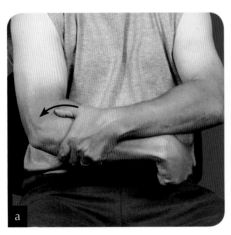

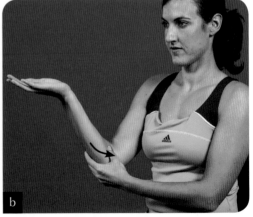

Figure 5.5 Direction of pressure when treating wrist extensors (a) and flexors (b).

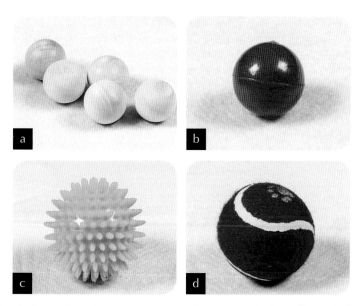

Figure 5.6   Balls used to direct pressure to soft tissues include golf-type balls *(a)*, high-bounce balls *(b)*, spikey therapy balls *(c)* or simple tennis-type balls *(d)*.

However, for many muscles using the thumb in this manner is not possible, so you may apply pressure to these muscle perpendicularly using a massage tool. In most cases this method is effective. Many tools are available to help create a lock. The easiest to use is a ball, such as a small golf-type ball or hard, high-bounce ball, a spikey therapy ball or simple tennis balls (see figure 5.6). Tennis balls have a tendency to split when pressed hard, so a good alternative is to use one of the tennis-type balls that are available as dog toys. They look like tennis balls but are much more firm and more durable.

One of the best tools to use for active STR is a dog ball on a rope (figure 5.7). The advantage of this tool will become apparent once you start to employ it to create locks when practicing active STR. Holding the rope prevents the ball dropping to the floor when using active STR in a standing position, for example.

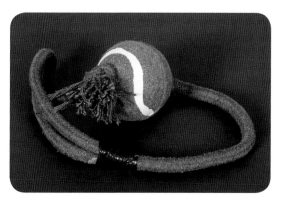

Figure 5.7   Dog ball on a rope.

Taking Up Slack in the Skin

Taking up slack in the skin prior to stretching results in a more effective stretch than when simply pressing into tissues. Unfortunately, taking up slack in the skin is only possible when applying active STR using thumbs; even then, it can be difficult to lock tissues sufficiently. The advantage of using active STR is that a client can use it independently every day. The advantage of passive and active-assisted STR is that slack can easily be taken up, creating a very effective stretch. It is often necessary to weigh up the advantages and disadvantages of each method of application and consider these factors in designing your treatment plan.

Incorporating Active-Assisted STR With Oil Massage

Incorporating STR with massage is most easily delivered by a therapist. Encourage clients to soothe an area after treatment with gentle rubbing, with or without a massage medium.

Active STR as Part of a Home Care Programme

Active STR is a useful technique to share with clients as part of their home care programme, and it is valuable as an adjunct to treatment. For example, if you are seeing a client once a week to try and resolve tension in the upper back and trapezius, passive or active-assisted STR can be highly beneficial. However, the client still has another 6 days during which to manage the condition. Many clients experience a relief from symptoms in the days following treatment, but by the end of the week symptoms have returned, especially if any aggravating factors have not been addressed. Working at a computer or driving for long periods of time where a static posture is maintained is a good example of how retention of a static posture might perpetuate symptoms. Providing clients with tips on applying STR on their own may help address the underlying condition and keep them engaged with their rehabilitation. In addition, many therapists find it useful to apply STR to their own forearms, which, even with good practice, often become excessively tight and develop trigger points.

Key Holds, Moves and Stances for Active STR

Illustrated here are 13 areas of the body that lend themselves to active STR: the plantar fascia on the sole of the foot, hamstrings, quadriceps, calf, gluteals, wrist and finger extensors and flexors, biceps brachii, trapezius, triceps, scalenes, rhomboids and pectorals. You can find detailed instructions for these stretches in chapters 6 through 8, where you can compare active STR to the passive and active-assisted techniques.

Foot

Sit down and place your foot on a tennis ball or spikey therapy ball with your ankle in neutral. Gently extend your toes, keeping your ankle in dorsiflexion. Work

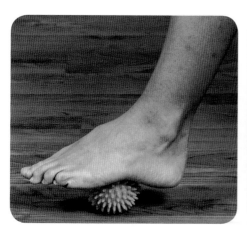
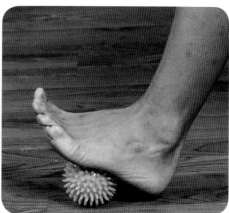

over the sole, moving the ball to discover which aspect of the fascia is tight and would benefit most from the stretch.

If giving this stretch as part of aftercare advice for a client, remember that it is not appropriate for people with diabetes, for example, who may have reduced sensation in the foot.

Hamstrings

Lie on your back, shorten the muscle by flexing your knee, and place a tennis ball over part of your hamstring muscles. Whilst holding the tennis ball as shown, gently extend your knee. Place your first lock (using the ball) near the ischium, and gradually work down towards your knee with subsequent locks.

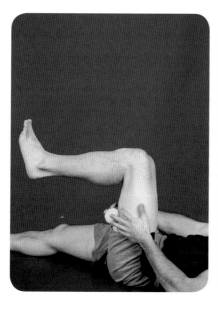
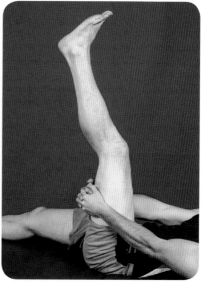

You can also apply active STR to the hamstrings in a seated position using a small ball placed between the thigh and a chair. With the ball in place, slowly extend the knee.

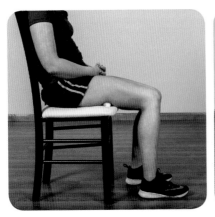 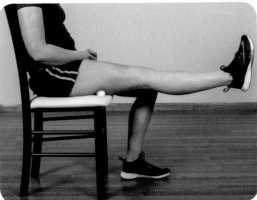

TIP For an interesting observation, use the straight-leg raise to test the length of the hamstrings, apply active STR either supine or seated, and then retest the length of the hamstrings. If active STR has been effective in reducing tension and lengthening tissues, you would expect the straight-leg raise to have changed and for there to be a greater degree of hip flexion.

Quadriceps

Whilst resting facedown, practise positioning the ball on various parts of your thigh; notice where you feel the most stretch. Position the ball first near your hip and work towards your knee with subsequent locks. For a slightly broader lock, you could use a roller like the one shown in figure 5.8.

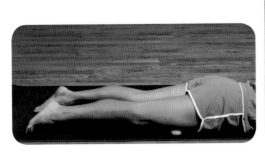 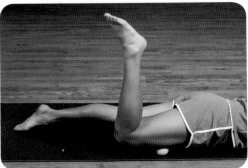

Calf

Resting on the floor with your legs straight in front of you, place your calf on a ball as shown in the photo. Gently dorsiflex your ankle to bring about the stretch. Again, for a slightly broader lock you could utilise a wooden roller (figure 5.8).

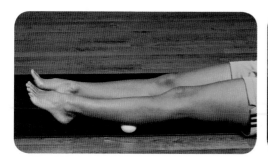 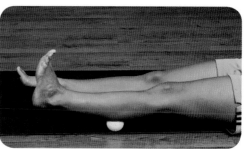

You could try this stretch in a seated position, resting your calf on a chair with the ball between your calf and the chair. However, you need to ensure that your leg is almost at the same height as the chair on which you are sitting in order to be able to apply STR over all of the calf.

TIP Before providing active STR to the calf for a client to do at home, remember to screen the client for contraindications such as varicose veins.

Gluteals

Although sitting on a tennis ball seems like a rational way to apply active STR to the gluteals, using the weight of the body can result in too much pressure being applied to one specific area. An alternative is to stand with your back to a wall, the ball between your buttock and the wall, then simply flex your hip.

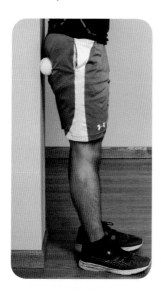 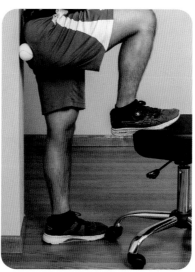

Wrist and Finger Extensors

Locate the bellies of your wrist and finger extensor muscles. Gently lock into the tissues with your wrist in extension. Take up the slack in soft tissues by pressing gently towards the elbow. Whilst maintaining your lock, gently flex your wrist. Work all over your wrist extensors from proximal (near the elbow) to distal (near the wrist).

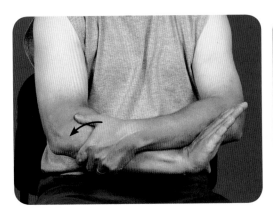 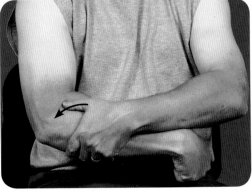

TIP You can more easily take up slack and achieve a lock if you apply a small amount of massage medium to the forearm, place a facecloth over the area you wish to treat, and press through the facecloth. The fronds in the cloth help provide grip, and the result is that you need less pressure to achieve the lock.

Another way to apply STR to the wrist extensors is to rest your forearms on a table with the palms facing upwards and use a small roller (figure 5.8) beneath the wrist extensors and the table. You may find that you need to use the hand of the forearm you are not treating to help stabilize the other forearm.

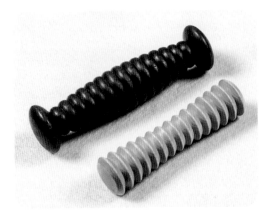

Figure 5.8 Wooden rollers can be useful for active STR.

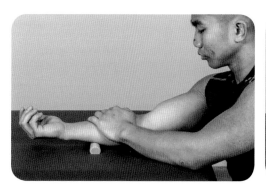 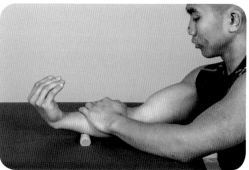

Wrist and Finger Flexors

Identify the bellies of your wrist and finger flexors. With your wrist in flexion, gently lock into this area, pulling the tissues gently towards the elbow. Whilst maintaining your lock, gently extend your wrist. Work your way from elbow to wrist. If providing this stretch for a client to use at home, remind the client that he or she does not need to press deeply into the wrist itself but can focus on the muscle bellies in the upper part of the forearm.

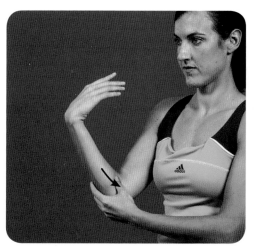 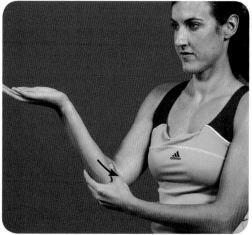

TIP As with active STR to the wrist extensors, working through a facecloth can make it easier to apply a lock.

Biceps Brachii

With your arm in flexion, gently grip your biceps muscle. Extend your elbow whilst maintaining your grip.

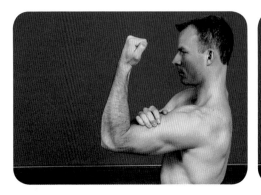 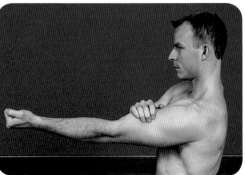

Triceps

To apply active STR to triceps, extend your arm and grip the muscle. Whilst maintaining your grip, gently flex your elbow.

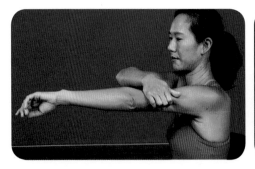 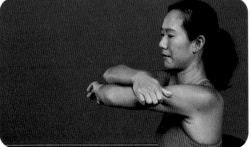

CLIENT TALK

A client sought treatment for pain in both upper arms, the right more than the left, which she experienced mostly whilst at work. She had full range of movement at the shoulder and elbow, but her triceps and biceps felt tender to touch. Her job was to manually polish furniture in a stately home, and she did so by resting on one hand, the elbow extended, and polishing vigorously using a cloth in the other hand. She was taught how to apply active STR to her own triceps and encouraged to do this at the end of the day to alleviate tension in this muscle.

Trapezius

It is possible to apply active STR to the trapezius by placing a ball between the upper back and a wall. However, tension in this muscle is often in the upper fibres, which are difficult to access when using a ball placed between you and a wall. An alternative approach is to create a lock by hooking into the upper fibres of trapezius using the end of a curved-handled umbrella.

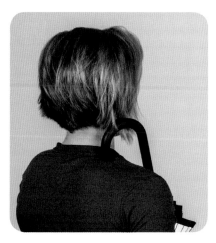 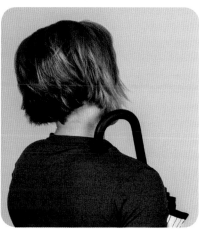

Scalenes

You can stretch the scalenes effectively using active STR. Using a finger only, apply gentle pressure just above the clavicle as you turn your head to the opposite direction. To treat the right scalenes, use the forefinger of your left hand and turn your head to the left. To treat the left scalenes, use the forefinger of your right hand and turn your head to the right. When teaching this technique to clients, instruct them to avoid pressing deeply into the front of the neck.

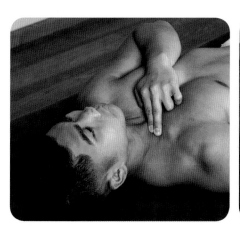 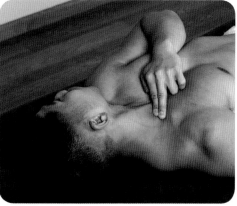

TIP Notice how you can achieve a greater stretch if you look up to the ceiling in addition to turning your head, and that you can move the jaw to enhance the stretch.

Rhomboids

To apply active STR to the rhomboid muscles it is necessary to place a ball between the rhomboids on one side of your back and the wall. Start with your hands by your sides, then bring about a stretch by flexing your shoulder and protracting your scapula. Repeat on the other side if necessary.

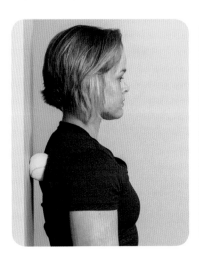 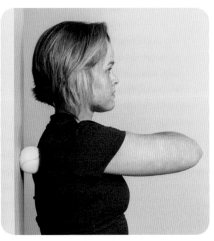

TIP As you move, the ball frequently drops to the floor unless you maintain pressure against the wall. One way to prevent the ball from dropping is to hold it inside a sock slung over your shoulder. Alternatively, you could use a ball on a rope.

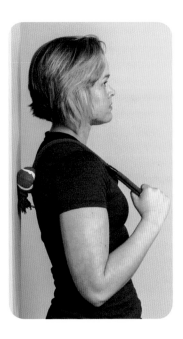

Pectorals

To apply active STR to pectorals, begin with your arm by your side. With the other hand, gently take up slack in the skin, drawing it towards the sternum; maintaining this lock, abduct your arm. The more you abduct, the greater the degree of stretch you achieve.

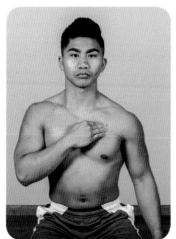 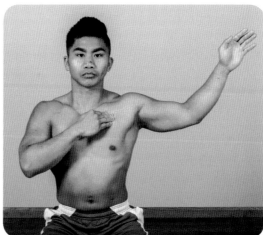

CLIENT TALK

A client's job involved manually unloading medium-sized parcels, which meant that he was constantly lifting parcels from pallets, carrying them short distances and re-stacking them onto shelves. Postural assessment revealed he had protracted scapulae and marginal kyphosis. He was advised to perform active STR for the pectoralis major at the end of his shift and to combine it with active chest stretches. He also received advice on the use of upper back strengthening exercises for postural correction.

Safety Guidelines for Active STR

Active STR is safe and effective. However, it is useful to be aware of certain cautions before practising this technique, especially because in some cases there may be quite a lot of pressure to body tissues.

- Avoid active STR if you have had a recent injury or if you bruise easily.

- When applying STR to the plantar fascia, do not transfer your whole body weight onto the tennis or therapy ball, and never try to stand on the ball as this could cause you to loose balance and fall.

- If you are using STR to self-treat plantar fasciitis or golfer's or tennis elbow, proceed with caution. Apply the technique gently for a maximum of 3 minutes. Most people will find active STR alleviates some of the discomfort of these conditions. However, if your condition seems aggravated within 12 hours of application, do not repeat STR. Avoid the use of active STR if you lack sensitivity in the area being treated.

- Do not use active STR to the sole of the foot if you have reduced sensation in the foot.

- Do not use active STR to the calf if you have varicose veins.

- Do not use active STR to the hamstrings if you have varicose veins in the back of the thigh.

- Active STR should not be used where osteoporosis is known or suspected.

- Be careful not to overwork any one area. Although soft tissue release is a great way to stretch muscles, stop after you have applied STR two or three times to one area. See how that area feels the next day. If it feels sore, do not repeat STR.

- Be careful when using STR to help lengthen the tissues acting on a joint that has been immobilized. Skin integrity may be compromised at this time. The skin may be particularly fragile if you have been in a plaster cast, for example.

- Avoid active deep STR before a sporting event. Whilst it may be tempting to use the technique to stretch out hamstrings before a race, for example, deep stretching should be avoided because it may decrease muscle power.

- Be careful when using your thumbs to lock into tissues, as in treating the wrist flexors and extensors. These muscles are relatively small, and little pressure is required to fix them during the stretch. If you discover that applying STR in this way starts to hurt your thumbs, have passive STR done for you or find an alternative method to lock the tissues.

When Is Active STR Indicated?

Active STR may be used directly through clothing all over the body as part of a general stretching routine. It is also useful for addressing trigger points; you may place a ball or massage tool over the point and apply pressure before the stretch.

Table 5.1 provides suggestions for when active treatment to particular muscles may be useful.

Table 5.1   Situations in Which Active STR Can Help

Muscle	Situation
Plantar fascia	<ul><li>To treat plantar fasciitis</li><li>After standing for long periods</li><li>After exercise, such as running or walking</li><li>To treat foot muscle cramps</li><li>To help regain flexibility in the plantar fascia after an injury such as an ankle sprain</li><li>To help regain flexibility in foot muscles after immobilization in a cast, such as with a ruptured Achilles tendon</li></ul>
Hamstrings	<ul><li>To treat tight hamstrings</li><li>After sitting for long periods</li><li>To increase knee extension after immobilization of the knee joint</li></ul>
Quadriceps	<ul><li>After exercise involving the quadriceps, such as walking, running or stepping</li><li>After standing for long periods</li></ul>
Calf	<ul><li>After exercise that uses the calf muscles a lot, such as tennis, running or basketball</li><li>After immobilization of the ankle</li></ul>
Wrist and finger extensors and flexors	<ul><li>For typists</li><li>For tennis players (extensors), golfers (flexors) and drivers (flexors)</li><li>After carrying heavy bags</li><li>For sports that require gripping, such as rock climbing or rowing</li><li>For massage therapists</li><li>After immobilization of the wrist or elbow</li></ul>
Biceps brachii	<ul><li>For any activity with prolonged or repetitive elbow flexion, such as rowing, digging or carrying</li><li>After immobilization of the elbow or shoulder</li></ul>
Triceps	<ul><li>For any activity involving prolonged or repetitive extension of the elbow, such as tennis</li><li>For massage therapists</li><li>After immobilization of the elbow or shoulder</li></ul>

Using Active STR to Treat Trigger Points

Active STR is an effective way to treat trigger points. One reason is that it is likely to be used more frequently than passive or active-assisted STR, which might otherwise only be delivered as part of a weekly treatment. Even where a client is not familiar with the concept of trigger points, most quickly learn how to identify them. When teaching a client how to identify trigger points, it is important to stress that pressure to the point should elicit slight discomfort but should not be painful. Because most clients are unlikely to have the same level of anatomical understanding as you do, advise them not to press into joints or onto bones or veins. It is also useful to explain that pressing a trigger point to the point of pain is counterproductive to the relaxation of muscles and that there is no place for the 'no-pain-no-gain' approach. Obviously, clients who are unwell or with injuries should avoid active STR unless they are themselves therapists and can identify contraindications.

When explaining to clients how to use active STR to treat trigger points, use these steps:

1. Shorten the muscle you intend to work on. Demonstrate this concept to the client using the muscle he or she plans to treat.

2. Show the client how to palpate the area to locate a trigger point. Self-palpation is not possible when working on the back of the body, so use a ball instead. When the client presses on the ball, moving his or her body over it, he or she should be able to locate trigger points.

3. Press gently over the point. It should feel slightly uncomfortable but not painful.

4. Maintaining the lock, gently lengthen the muscle, stretching the fibres.

5. Release your lock and soothe the area.

6. Feel for the trigger point again, and repeat the technique a total of three or four times.

Wherever possible, use passive or active-assisted STR on a trigger point so that your client has an understanding of the sensation and the process involved. Explain to your client that as the trigger point dissipates it will become more difficult to locate and feel less (if at all) uncomfortable when pressed. Trigger points rarely disappear with a single treatment session but will resolve with time. Importantly, a client should keep a mental or written note about his or her experiences of using active STR to treat trigger points. That way, you can help address any errors and identify why active STR is or is not working in deactivation of trigger points.

How to Become Proficient in the Use of Active STR

See table 5.2 for an overview of active STR applications. The following points will help you to get the most out of your practice sessions:

- Practise using different tools to lock tissues. Compare using a tennis ball to using a dog ball, for example.
- Identify which parts of your body are hard to access even when using a tool and which may therefore benefit from passive or active-assisted STR.
- Practise applying a massage medium. Use oil or wax, placing a facecloth over the area, then creating a lock. This works especially well on wrist extensors.
- Identify any locks that feel uncomfortable, and ask yourself why it might be so. Is it the position you need to adopt, or is it the method of locking that causes discomfort?
- Practise at least two times on each of the muscles.

Quick Questions

1. How do I shorten the muscle I want to work on?
2. Do I contract first and then lock, or lock and then contract?
3. How do I know which way to work along the muscle?
4. Can I use STR if I bruise easily?
5. For how long can I apply active STR to one muscle?

Table 5.2 Overview of Active STR Applications

Foot	Hamstrings		Quadriceps
Seated Ball	Supine Ball	Seated Ball	Prone Ball

Calf	Gluteals	Wrist and finger extensors	
Supine Ball	Standing Ball	Seated Thumb	Seated Roller

Wrist and finger flexors	Biceps brachii	Triceps	Upper trapezius
Seated Thumb	Seated Grip	Seated Grip	Seated Curved handle of umbrella

Scalenes	Rhomboids	Pectorals
Supine Fingertips	Standing Ball	Seated Fingertips

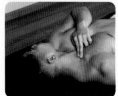 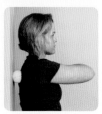 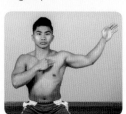

Applying Soft Tissue Release

The three chapters in part III provide detailed information about how to apply STR to various muscles of the body. In chapter 6 you will learn how to apply STR to these muscles of the trunk: rhomboids, pectorals, levator scapulae, upper fibres of the trapezius, erector spinae and scalenes. Chapter 7 focuses on these muscles of the lower limbs: hamstrings, calf, foot, quadriceps, tibialis anterior, fibulari (peroneals), gluteals, iliotibial band (ITB) and iliacus. Chapter 8 provides examples of how to apply STR to these muscles of the upper limbs: triceps, biceps brachii, shoulder adductors, infraspinatus, and wrist and finger flexors and extensors.

Each chapter begins with an overview in the form of a table enabling you to quickly identify the muscles contained in that chapter and which forms of STR can be used for them.

Within each chapter are illustrations of each of the muscles showing common sites of trigger points, with text describing where they refer pain, how to locate them and what perpetuates these points. Where available, references relating to the deactivation of trigger points are provided. Photographs showing start and end positions are provided along with detailed step-by-step guidelines, plus the advantages and disadvantages of each stretch. For most of the muscles there are descriptions and photographs of how STR can be applied in these treatment positions: prone, supine, side lying, seated or standing. The chapters include plenty of helpful tips and some Client Talk boxes, with examples of how some of the stretches have been used in real-life situations. As usual, chapters end with Quick Questions with which to test yourself. Use these chapters in any order to help you master all three types of STR.

Soft Tissue Release for the Trunk

This chapter outlines how to apply soft tissue release to the trunk. You will find comparisons between applying passive, active-assisted and active STR to each of the major muscle groups of the trunk. You will also find illustrations showing key trigger points in each muscle. As with chapters 3, 4 and 5, this chapter includes a table providing an overview of the techniques for each muscle; in this case, it shows whether the technique illustrated is passive, active-assisted or active (table 6.1).

Table 6.1   Types of STR Used on Trunk Muscles

Muscle	Passive	Active-assisted	Active
Rhomboids	✓	–	✓
Pectorals	✓	✓	✓
Levator scapulae	–	✓	–
Upper trapezius	–	✓	✓
Erector spinae (spinalis)	–	✓	–
Scalenes	–	✓	✓

■   *Passive STR:* It is useful to apply STR passively to the rhomboids and pectorals. However, when working with tissues of the neck, active-assisted STR is a more appropriate method of application. Active-assisted STR puts the client in charge of his or her own neck movements and therefore the degree of stretch received.

■   *Active-assisted STR:* This technique is a useful method of safely stretching the pectorals, levator scapulae, upper trapezius, erector spinae and scalenes. It may be used on the rhomboids, but with the client in the prone position, these muscles are quickly fatigued. Applying active-assisted STR to the rhomboids also makes it difficult for the therapist to firmly lock the tissues, which are relatively small and shorten when concentrically contracted. For these reasons, illustrations of active-assisted STR to the rhomboids have not been included here.

- *Active STR:* Whilst trunk muscles are often included in an overall stretching routine, these muscles are generally not stretched using active STR, because it is fairly difficult to lock the tissues correctly without causing strain to other body parts.

The following section provides detailed instructions for applying passive, active-assisted or active STR to many of the muscles of the trunk, including tips that may help you apply these techniques. Advantages and disadvantages of each application are also included.

Trigger Points in the Rhomboids

Trigger points in the rhomboid muscles (figure 6.1) cause pain in the rhomboid area but can also cause symptoms in the region of the supraspinatus. The best way to palpate rhomboid muscles to locate trigger points is with the shoulder flexed and the scapula protracted. The application of STR to the rhomboid muscles lends itself well to the identification of trigger points as, whether STR is performed with the client prone (passive STR), seated (active-assisted STR), or standing (active STR), the scapula can be protracted. You can find trigger points throughout the rhomboid muscles between the medial border of the scapula and the spine. In many people, the

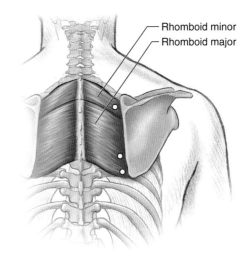

Figure 6.1 Trigger points in the rhomboid muscles.

rhomboids are lengthened and weak, so whilst STR *can* be applied to them, it is important to ask yourself whether it *should* be applied to them. Before you begin, note whether your client has a kyphotic posture, the posture associated with protraction of the scapulae with stretched and weak rhomboids. If you are not sure how assess the client's posture, refer to a text such as *Postural Assessment* (Johnson, 2012).

When treating a client with a typical thoracic curve, you may apply STR to trigger points by following any of the methods (passive, active-assisted or active). Locate the trigger points and, whilst maintaining your lock, stretch the tissues. Clients with active trigger points in the rhomboid muscles often also have active points in the upper fibres of trapezius too, so to be fully effective it is important to deactivate those trigger points. If your client has a kyphotic posture, then trigger points can be deactivated through gentle pressure, but avoid overstretching the muscles afterwards. Instead, encourage your client to engage in a programme for strengthening the rhomboids and the lower fibres of trapezius.

Tewari et al. (2017) report how they deactivated two trigger points in the left rhomboids and left erector spinae of a person with Ehlers-Danlos syndrome (a form of hypermobility) who had chronic upper-back pain. They injected the triggers with lignocaine, and they prescribed the application of heat and 10 minutes of deep massage twice a day. Seven days later, the subject reported a 60 to 80 percent relief from pain, which had been measured using a visual analogue scale (VAS).

Botha (2017) compared ischaemic compression with the use of a foam roller for the deactivation of trigger points in the rhomboid muscle; 30 participants were randomly split into either the compression or foam roller group. Six treatments were delivered over a period of 6 weeks, and both subjective (questionnaire and VAS) and objective (pressure algometer) measurements were taken. Botha concluded that both treatments were equally effective at reducing trigger points with neither being superior.

Passive STR for Rhomboids: Prone

Step 1: Position your client in the prone position on a treatment couch so that he or she is able to flex at the shoulder. To do so you will need to position your client so that the arm can hang off the couch. A safe approach is to have the client lie at an angle on the couch, feet positioned at the corner opposite to the arm you are working on. With your client in this position, shorten the rhomboids by passively retracting the scapula, holding the client's arm just above the elbow (figure 6.2*a*). It does not matter whether the client rests the head to the left or to the right, as long as he or she is comfortable.

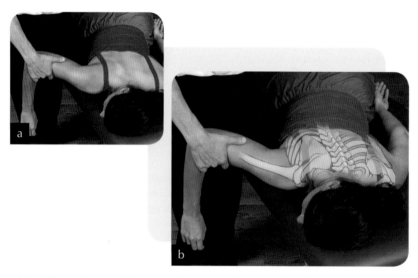

Figure 6.2 Lifting the arm *(a)* passively retracts the scapula, bringing it closer to the spine *(b)*.

Step 2: Whilst holding the client's arm to keep the rhomboids passively shortened, gently lock the tissues, directing your pressure towards the spine (figure 6.3). As you can see from figure 6.2*b,* the ribs curve outward. It is therefore important to direct your pressure towards the spine rather than perpendicularly, because pressing into the ribs would be uncomfortable for the client.

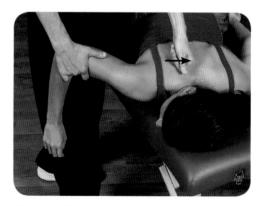

Figure 6.3 Directing pressure towards the spine.

Step 3: Whilst maintaining your lock and still pressing gently towards the spine, gently lower your client's arm into flexion (figure 6.4*a*). Notice how the scapula protracts around the rib cage (figure 6.4*b*), stretching the rhomboids.

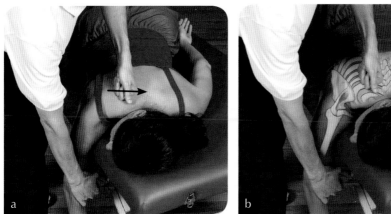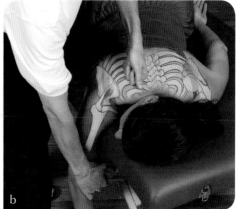

Figure 6.4   Passively flexing the arm *(a)* protracts the scapula around the rib cage *(b)*.

Relatively speaking, the rhomboids are a small group of muscles and cannot be worked in lines running between their insertion point as some other muscles can. Change the position of your lock to any point on the rhomboids as you repeat the procedure. To deactivate trigger points here, use your thumb or fingers to gently depress the trigger prior to the stretch.

TIP   You may need to practise repositioning your client to ensure flexion at the shoulder. If the client is not correctly positioned, this technique may cause pressure on the brachial plexus in the armpit, which could be uncomfortable, sometimes causing temporary numbness or tingling in the fingers that lasts until the client is repositioned.

If you find using your fist uncomfortable for your wrist, try using your forearm for the lock. This area is bony, so use elbows with caution.

Whilst it is possible to use active-assisted STR with your client in this position, it is a little tricky; the client needs to retract and protract his or her own scapula, which can be tiring. Also, you need to take care where you stand so as to be out of the way of the client's moving arm. Standing at the head of the couch, rather than to the side, is one solution. From this position you can use reinforced fingers to lock the tissues.

CLIENT TALK

Active-assisted STR to the rhomboids in prone was particularly useful when treating a female rower with large musculature. By combining this technique with lots of oil massage, it was possible to get good leverage on the client's muscles and I used my elbow to localise the stretch to specific areas of tightness. However, it was necessary to work through a facecloth, because it was quite difficult to get a firm enough lock on the skin alone.

Advantages
- You have considerable leverage and will be able to fix the muscles well.
- Working with the scapula protracted means you can access the rhomboids well and this is especially useful when treating trigger points.

Disadvantages
- If the client is not correctly positioned, this technique may cause uncomfortable pressure on the brachial plexus in the armpit.
- Use of inappropriate posture when lifting and lowering the client's arm could cause you to hurt your back.
- This technique cannot easily be incorporated into an oil massage because it requires the client to be positioned diagonally on the treatment couch, which would mean moving the client several times during treatment.
- With good leverage, some therapists accidentally press too hard; it is especially uncomfortable when working over ribs.
- Unless your client is engaged in regular physical activity, it may be unlikely he or she needs the rhomboids stretched. Many clients have kyphotic postures, with protracted shoulders. When the shoulders are protracted, the rhomboids are lengthened. Do you need to stretch them further?

Passive STR for Rhomboids: Seated

Step 1: With your client comfortably seated, gently hold his or her arm to passively retract the scapula, shortening the rhomboids. Take up the slack in the skin, directing your pressure towards the spine (figure 6.5a). You may need to practise different handholds, sometimes supporting the client's forearm on yours, in order to help him or her relax and give you the weight of the arm. With the scapula retracted, you have little space to position your lock (figure 6.5b), so you may need several attempts before both you and your client are comfortable.

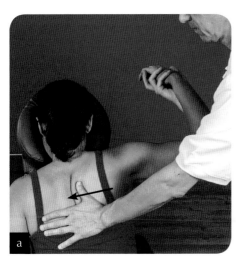
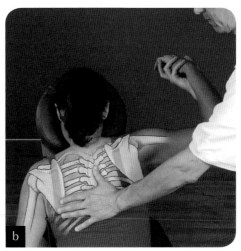

Figure 6.5 Taking up slack in the skin *(a)* as the scapula is passively retracted, moving it closer to the spine and shortening the rhomboids *(b)*.

Step 2: Whilst maintaining your lock, take the arm into flexion, which passively protracts the scapula (figure 6.6).

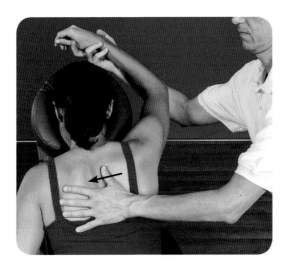

Figure 6.6 Passively protracting the scapula.

If you wish to use STR to deactivate trigger points in the rhomboids, it is easiest to palpate the muscles whilst the scapula is protracted. To facilitate this position, ask your client to hug him- or herself, freeing up both of your hands to locate the trigger points. You can then return to performing passive STR as described.

TIP One way to make this process easier for yourself is to apply a little oil to the area and then ask your client to put on an old T-shirt. Apply STR through the T-shirt, which will help facilitate your lock.

Advantages

- In this position, you have less leverage and are therefore less likely to apply too much pressure. As a result, it is a good method of working with clients who are especially sensitive to pressure.
- It is also helpful when working with clients who cannot lie in the prone position.

Disadvantages

- Locking the tissues using your thumb risks injury to the joint in the thumb. This risk can be lessened by restricting the use of the technique and using only light pressure.
- It is difficult to perform passive STR on clients with long or heavy limbs.
- Some clients find it difficult to relax during passive STR and will always tense their limbs.
- When the client is sitting, the muscles of the posterior trunk are not as relaxed as in prone.

It is possible to use active-assisted STR to the rhomboids with your client seated. However, to do so you need to stand directly behind the client in order to be out of the way of the arm as he or she horizontally flexes and extends the shoulder. Standing directly behind the client in this way makes it difficult to press the soft tissues over the rhomboids towards the spine, which is necessary in order to take up slack at the start of the technique.

Active STR for Rhomboids: Standing

Step 1: Stand with your back close to a wall. Place a ball on a rope or another kind of small, hard ball, between your upper back and the wall, over the area of the rhomboids (figure 6.7). If using this method to teach clients how to use active STR, be certain to advise them that they should avoid pressure to the spine. The dorsal scapular nerve runs parallel to the medial border of the scapula, so you should avoid deep pressure here.

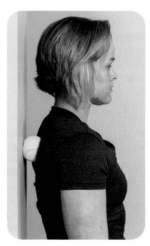

Figure 6.7 Positioning a ball between the rhomboids and a wall.

Step 2: Start with your arm by your side. Reposition the ball if necessary to get it into the correct place over the rhomboids. When you are happy that the ball is in the correct position, horizontally flex your shoulder, and protract the scapula (figure 6.8).

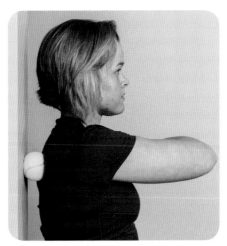

Figure 6.8   Protracting the scapula to stretch the rhomboids.

Advantage

- Active STR can be practised anywhere there is a wall. Therefore, it is likely to be effective for deactivating trigger points as it can be performed frequently.

Disadvantages

- Repeating active STR too many times, or pressing too deeply, can cause soreness.

- The technique is not suitable for anyone with osteoporosis or for whom pressure to the posterior rib cage might cause problems.

CLIENT TALK

I taught a client how to actively use STR to treat his rhomboid muscles. They were tight and sore due to his job, which involved carrying long planks of wood from where they were delivered by crane, to where they needed to be sawn for furniture making. To carry the wood the client balanced it on his shoulder, one plank at a time, using one arm in front of him and one behind him to support the plank. Imagine you are carrying wood in this way, and notice how you need to retract the scapula of the arm that you take behind you. Providing the client with this technique meant he could use it daily to alleviate pain.

Trigger Points in the Pectorals

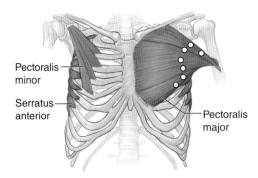

Figure 6.9   Trigger points in pectoralis major and pectoralis minor.

Trigger points develop throughout pectoralis major. Shown in figure 6.9 are those in the clavicular, sternal and lateral portions of the muscle. The clavicular portion refers pain locally to that part of the muscle as well as to the anterior deltoid. The sternal portion refers pain to the anterior chest on that side, as well as down the arm on that side, especially to the medial epicondyle. When severe, pain can radiate to the little and ring finger on that side also. Finally, the lateral portion has trigger points located in the front aspect of the axilla and can cause breast sensitivity or pain.

Trigger points found in the upper and lower portions of pectoralis minor refer pain to the anterior deltoid primarily, the chest and the anteromedial side of the arm. Trigger points in pectoralis minor increase the tonicity of this muscle and cause protrusion of the inferior angle of the scapula due to pulling of the muscle on the coracoid process, which tilts the scapula anteriorly. Tension in this muscle also causes the scapula to rotate and is a major cause of scapulothoracic dysfunction, affecting movement of the shoulder and impairing performance in sporting populations.

Shortening of pectoralis major, if prolonged, can aggravate trigger points. This muscle is shortened in clients with round-shouldered posture. Weakness in the rhomboids and the middle and lower fibres of trapezius is common in such a posture, causing trigger points to develop in those muscles also due to stretch weakness. Pain due to trigger points in pectoralis major reduces motion at the shoulder. Trigger points in pectoralis minor may be established and perpetuated by trigger points in the scalenes, poor posture, and, being muscles of respiration, by dysfunctional breathing such as forced or prolonged inspiratory effort.

To palpate trigger points in pectoralis major, position your client supine with the arm abducted to around 90 degrees. With the flat of your fingertips, work along the fibres of the muscle, starting with the clavicular portion and changing direction to match the change in direction of fibres. Trigger points in the lateral portion are easier to palpate if you gently pinch the front of the axilla between your finger and thumb. Palpation of trigger points in pectoralis minor is best achieved by passively shortening pectoralis major. Do so by abducting the client's arm whilst they rest in the supine position, and place a pillow or rolled up towel beneath it. Then, you can locate trigger points in the upper part of pectoralis minor by first identifying the coracoid process and feeling for the muscle attachment. You can identify lower triggers by gently squeezing the pectoralis major muscle between your finger and thumb, your thumb over pectoralis major. Active elevation of the shoulder in this position will cause pectoralis to become tensioned, making it easier to identify.

Research into the use of trigger point deactivation in pectoralis major has focused on clinical outcomes following mastectomy. Shin et al. (2014) examined the effectiveness of ultrasound-guided needling to trigger points in pectoralis major and infraspinatus in 19 post-mastectomy patients who each had shoulder pain and restricted movement of the shoulder on the surgical side. Additionally, all participants were instructed to stretch 20 times during the day, although which stretch was performed is not stated. VAS scores and shoulder range of movement improved immediately after the first injection and 3 months after the last injection compared to baseline measurements. In a case report, Cummings (2003) provides a detailed and interesting description of a patient who presented at the British Medical Acupuncture Society's London teaching clinic with a 5-month history of arm pain radiating down the ulnar side of the forearm, right to the fourth and fifth digits. A discrete area of tenderness was identified in the lateral portion of pectoralis major, which the author took to be a trigger point; however, the author notes that symptoms could be derived from both this and neuropathic pain from surgical damage to the intercostobrachial nerve. Some pain was resolved immediately after the first session of needling, and as all symptoms were resolved 2 weeks later; no further acupuncture was performed. Again, a home stretching programme was advised.

Use the STR techniques provided in this section to learn how to apply STR to most clients, especially for those with round-shouldered postures. If you want to use STR to treat trigger points, you will need to use a finger to locate and compress the point. For clients who report shoulder or arm pain following mastectomy where you have identified an active trigger, consider using gentle ischaemic compression, or gentle compression with mild stretch as is achieved with STR.

Passive STR for Pectoralis Major: Supine

Step 1: With your client in supine, take his or her arm into horizontal flexion and fix the tissues with a soft fist, directing your pressure towards the sternum rather than into the underlying ribs (figure 6.10). You may want to explain to your client where you are going to position your fist for the lock, because some clients may find it invasive.

TIP If you find it tricky to apply your lock, cushion the lock by working through a facecloth folded into fourths. Applying a little massage medium first will help the cloth grip the skin and facilitate the taking up of slack.

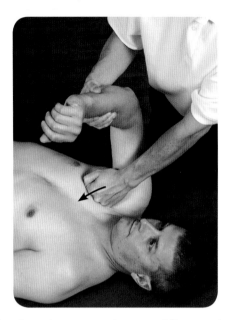

Figure 6.10 Passively taking the arm into horizontal flexion, shortening the pectoralis major muscle.

Step 2: Whilst maintaining your lock, gently take your client's arm from horizontal flexion into a more neutral position (figure 6.11).

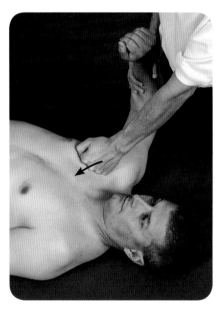

Figure 6.11 Passively extending the shoulder whilst maintaining the soft lock.

As you can see from figures 6.10 and 6.11, the movement is small, requiring only a subtle change in arm position for the client to experience this stretch. When treating a female client, you will need to focus on the upper fibres of pectoralis major and avoid working through breast tissue. When treating male clients, you may work over a greater part of the muscle.

TIP Avoid pressing downward into the ribs. If your fists are too large for the small area on which you need to work, try using the pads of your fingers and gently reinforce one hand over the other.

Some clients do not feel the stretch immediately. In this case, you must practise the technique by applying your pressure from various angles and stretching the tissues by moving the client's arm in varying degrees of abduction. However, clients with kyphotic postures may feel the stretch immediately because they have shortened pectorals.

Advantage

- This technique is relatively easy to incorporate into a holistic massage treatment.

Disadvantages

- It takes practice to direct pressure towards the sternum rather than downward into the ribs.
- Your hands may be too large to use your fists, especially if the client has a small frame. In this case, use your fingers but exercise care because there will be an increased likelihood of pressing into the ribs.
- It takes practice to know at which angle to abduct the arm, and the angle needed to facilitate the stretch varies considerably between clients.
- This stretch cannot be applied easily to clients with large breasts.
- It can be difficult finding the correct method of supporting the upper limb when working with larger clients.
- Clients with large and well-developed pectorals are unlikely to feel passive STR to the pectorals; a considerably stronger lock is required to fix the tissues of these clients.

Active-Assisted STR for Pectoralis Major: Supine

Step 1: Ask your client to move his or her arm across the body, which actively shortens the pectoralis major. Using soft fists, lock the muscle and direct your pressure towards the sternum (figure 6.12).

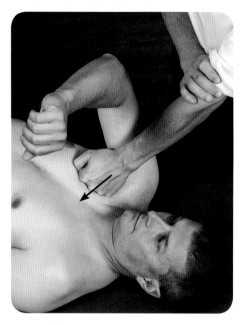

Figure 6.12 Active shortening of pectoralis major as the therapist gently locks the tissues.

Step 2: Whilst maintaining your lock, ask your client to move the arm so that he or she can feel the stretch in the pectorals. The client will need to move the arm from horizontal flexion into a more neutral position (figure 6.13).

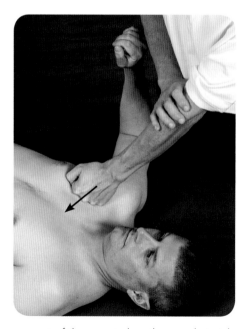

Figure 6.13 Active movement of the arm to lengthen and stretch pectoralis major.

Step 3: Release, and repeat steps 1 and 2 three times on each side of the body.

As with passive STR for pectoralis major, if you wish to deactivate trigger points in this muscle you will need to create your lock using a finger.

Advantages

- The client will be able to locate the precise position where he or she feels the stretch.
- You can reinforce the lock using two soft fists or reinforced fingers.

Disadvantage

- It can be tricky at first to find the best place to stand as the client moves his or her arm in search of the stretch. However, once the client finds the position, the treatment can proceed without disruption.

Active STR for Pectorals: Seated or Standing

Step 1: With your arm by your side, seated or standing, gently draw the skin and soft tissues of your chest towards your sternum (figure 6.14). It can be difficult to lock tissues through clothing, slightly easier without clothing, and easiest of all if you apply a little massage medium and then lock the tissues through a cloth or an old T-shirt.

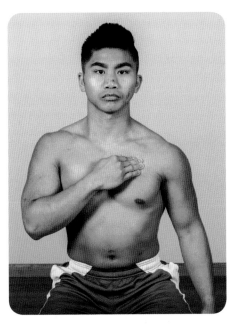

Figure 6.14 Locking the tissues of the chest for active STR.

Step 2: Maintaining your lock, gently abduct and extend your arm, producing a stretch (figure 6.15). Practise changing to the position of your arm to discover where you best feel the stretch.

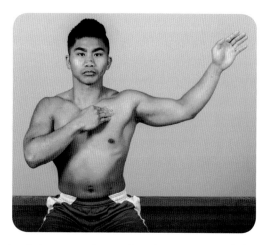

Figure 6.15 Actively abducting and extending the arm to stretch the tissues in active STR.

To deactivate trigger points in the lateral portion of the pectoralis muscle, gently pinch the front of your armpit, palpating until you locate a trigger point. Maintain your grip, then abduct and extend your arm. To deactivate trigger points in the rest of the muscle, gently roll a firm ball over the muscle until you locate a trigger point. Hold the ball in place as you abduct and extend your arm. For example, to treat a trigger in the left pectoralis muscle, press the ball gently over the point using your right hand as you move your left arm to create the stretch.

Trigger Points in the Levator Scapulae

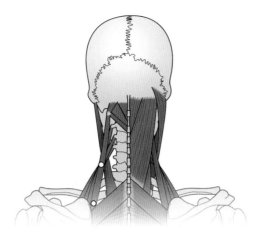

Figure 6.16 Trigger points in the levator scapulae.

Trigger points found in the levator scapulae (figure 6.16) produce pain locally and down the medial border of the scapula as well as to the back of the shoulder. When active, these trigger points can limit rotation of the neck and cause feelings of neck stiffness. Many factors perpetuate these points, including carrying a bag on one shoulder, retaining a static posture with the head turned slightly to one side, using a walking aid that is too high and which causes the user to walk with the shoulder elevated, as well as repetitive overhead actions of the arm. Trigger points in the levator scapulae are relatively easy to identify. The easiest point to identify is the inferior of the two, which is found close to the insertion of the muscle on the superior angle of the scapula. The more superior point can be found at the point where the levator scapulae can be palpated independent of the anterior border of the upper fibres of the trapezius.

TIP To make palpation of these triggers easier, work with the upper fibres of the trapezius in a passively shortened position. For example, if palpating your client in a seated position, support his or her arm on a table; if working with the client in a prone position, place a small towel beneath the shoulder on that side; when palpating in the side-lying position, position the uppermost arm in such a way as to reduce depression of the shoulder. The upper trigger point can also be palpated when the client is supine and the trapezius is relaxed.

In a randomized clinical trial, De Meulemeester et al. (2017) compared trigger point dry needling with manual pressure for the deactivation of trigger points in 42 female office workers who each did a minimum of 20 hours of computer work per week and who each had myofascial neck or shoulder pain. Baseline measurements were taken using a numerical rating scale, the Neck Disability Index

(NDI), pressure pain thresholds and muscle characteristics. Six trigger points were identified for treatment, including those in the levator scapulae, and participants were treated once a week for four weeks. At the end of the study, no significant differences existed between the groups; both resulted in a significant improvement in NDI scores. Significant improvements also occurred in the other outcomes of pain, muscle elasticity and stiffness.

The active-assisted method of applying STR described in this section is an ideal way to help deactivate trigger points in the levator scapulae. For best effect, you will most likely need to deactivate trigger points in the scalenes and posterior cervical muscles, as these too restrict movement and can inhibit full release of the levator scapulae.

Applying STR to the levator scapulae is particularly useful when treating clients with a stiff neck or shoulder problems. It is safe to use on the neck area because the stretch is performed actively, within the client's comfort level, making it unlikely that the tissues would ever be overstretched.

Active-Assisted STR for Levator Scapulae: Seated

Step 1: Locate the levator scapulae by gently palpating up the medial border of the scapula to the insertion point of the muscle on this bone (figure 6.17a). Note that you will be close to, if not on a trigger point in this region (figure 6.17b), so press gently as it can be tender.

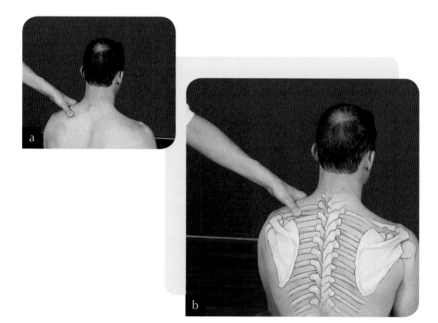

Figure 6.17 Identifying the levator scapulae by palpating up the medial border of the scapula (a) to the superior angle (b).

Step 2: Lock the muscle (figure 6.18). The levator scapulae is a strap-like muscle and is often hypertonic (extremely tight), yet long in people with forward-head postures and those who are prone to weakness.

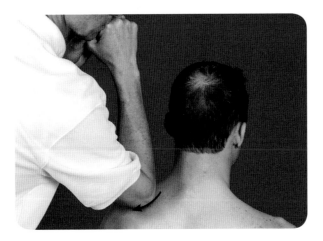

Figure 6.18   Gently locking the levator scapulae using an elbow.

Step 3: Whilst maintaining your lock, ask your client to rotate the head to about 45 degrees and then lower the chin to look to the floor (figure 6.19). Repeat the movement three times and then apply the same stretch to the opposite side of the body.

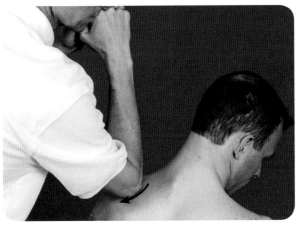

Figure 6.19   The client performs the stretch by flexing and rotating the head away from the therapist.

TIP This muscle is so hypertonic in many clients that they cannot tolerate a stretch at all; simply locking the muscle provides some relief for their tension. If you find this to be the case, use gentle ischaemic compression to reduce the trigger points, address trigger points in the scalenes and erector spinae, and then return to the levator scapulae.

CLIENT TALK

I taught two telephonists how to perform active-assisted STR. They used it gently in treating each other, taking turns throughout the day, in order to alleviate tension in each other's neck muscles.

Advantages

- When you work in this position, you have easy access to the muscle and good leverage.
- There is little danger that soft tissues of the neck will be overstretched, because the client is in charge of the stretch. Provided that the client is reminded to stretch only within a comfortable, pain-free range, this technique should always be a safe way to use STR to stretch this muscle.

Disadvantages

- This muscle is so hypertonic in many clients that they cannot tolerate a stretch.
- For the stretch to be really effective, it is essential to show the client specifically where to move the head once you have locked the tissues; otherwise, there is a tendency for them to flex the neck without also rotating it, and this lessens the effectiveness of the stretch.
- Make sure that for each new lock, the client's neck is in neutral, with the head facing forward. If you place your lock when the neck is in slight flexion, it lessens the effectiveness of the stretch.

Trigger Points in the Upper Trapezius

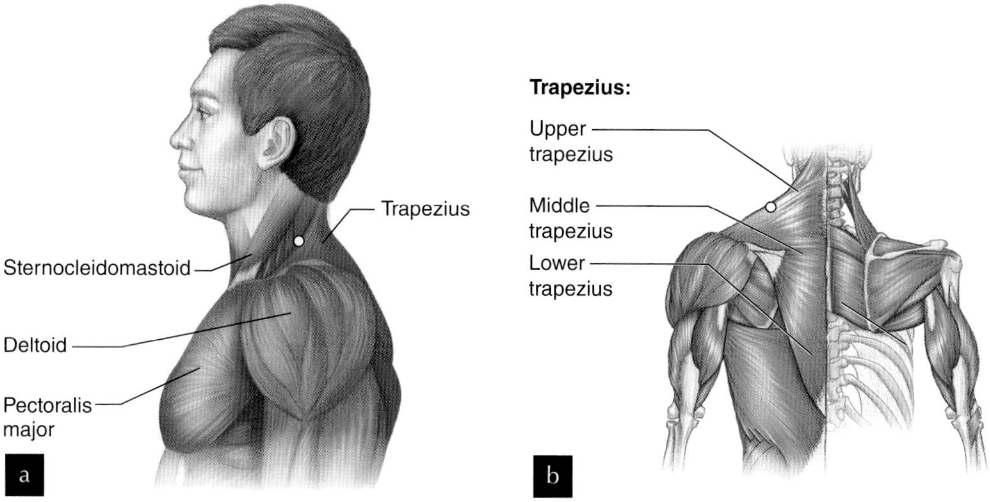

Figure 6.20 Trigger points in the upper trapezius; side view (a) and back view (b).

Trigger points are found in the upper, middle and lower fibres of the trapezius. In this section you will discover how you can utilise STR to help deactivate those in the upper fibres. In the side view (figure 6.20a) you can see the trigger point that refers pain to the side of the neck, head, eye and jaw. This trigger is located around midway in the anterior fibres of the muscle and contributes to symptoms associated with tension headache. It is more likely when trigger points are in suboccipital temporal and the sternocleidomastoid muscles, so all muscles should be treated for trigger points when attempting to reduce headache that is of muscular origin. Trigger points in the upper fibres of the trapezius (see figure 6.20) can develop from carrying a heavy bag on one shoulder; a rucksack; tight bra straps pressing into the muscle; trauma such as whiplash associated disorders (WAD); lower limb discrepancy, which causes lateral curvature of the spine; and uneven shoulder height resulting in overactivity of the upper fibres on one side to maintain head position. Sitting with one arm passively raised, as is common when some people drive and rest an arm on an open window side of the car door, and repetitive overarm movement from sports or hobbies both contribute to the perpetuation of active trigger points. Conversely, tension from prolonged lack of support when using the arms can also aggravate triggers.

You can locate the trigger points in the upper fibres of the trapezius by gently pinching the upper fibres between your finger and thumb and exploring them to find the tender point. Passive elevation of the arm can make this task easier, as can palpation of the client in a supine position. Try this technique on your own muscle: sit with your right arm supported on the arm rest of a chair or table and your right shoulder slightly elevated. Using the forefinger and thumb of your left hand, gently pinch the upper portion of your right trapezius, rolling it beneath your forefinger until you locate the point.

Moraska et al. (2017) examined the responsiveness of trigger points to single and multiple trigger point release massages to the upper trapezius muscle in 62 people with tension-type headache. Participants were randomly assigned to one of these three groups: a wait list where no treatment was prescribed, a sham ultrasound group, or a group receiving ischaemic compression of trigger points bilaterally in the upper trapezius and suboccipital. Treatment was provided twice-weekly for 6 weeks and lasted 45 minutes and in the massage group trapezius was treated by gripping the muscle between the thumb and finger whilst the participant was supine. Using an algometer, pressure pain threshold was measured at baseline and after the first and twelfth treatments. They found that the pressure pain threshold increased after both the first and twelfth treatment in the massage group only.

In a study of 45 volunteers, Taleb, Youssef and Saleh (2016) explored the effectiveness of manual versus algometer pressure release techniques in active trigger points in the upper trapezius. The pressure pain threshold and active side bending of the head were assessed at baseline and after treatment. Results revealed that participants who had received trigger point release with the algometer had a significant increase in the side-bending range, which the authors suggest may be due to the consistency of pressure delivered when using the device.

Active-Assisted STR for Upper Trapezius: Seated

Step 1: With your client sitting, lock the upper fibres of the trapezius (figure 6.21).

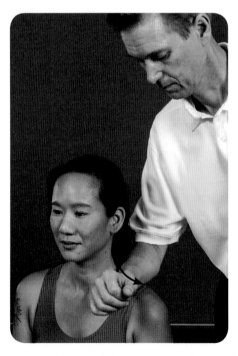

Figure 6.21 Locking the upper fibres of the trapezius using the forearm.

Step 2: Whilst maintaining your lock, ask your client to laterally flex the neck until feeling a comfortable stretch (figure 6.22).

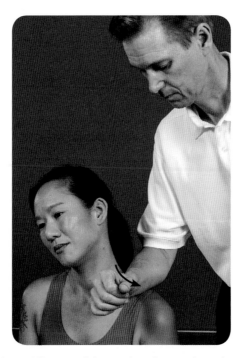

Figure 6.22   Active lateral flexion of the neck to bring about the stretch.

Step 3: Repeat the action three times, then repeat the same stretch on the opposite side of the body.

Advantages

- When you work in this position, you have easy access to the muscle and good leverage.
- There is little danger that soft tissues of the neck will be overstretched, because the client is in charge of the stretch. Provided that the client is reminded to stretch only within a comfortable, pain-free range, this technique should always be a safe way to use STR to stretch this muscle.
- With practice, and by working with the client, you will be able to alter the direction of pressure to localize the stretch to different fibres in the upper trapezius.

Disadvantage

- It is easy to press into bony structures, such as the clavicle and acromion process.

Active-Assisted STR for Upper Trapezius: Supine

Using active-assisted STR with the client in the supine position is a good way to deactivate trigger points in the upper fibres of trapezius.

Step 1: With your client in the supine position, palpate for trigger points. If treating trigger points in the anterior fibres, gently lock the tissues using your thumb or a massage tool (figure 6.23). To treat the posterior trigger in the upper trapezius, use a firm ball, getting feedback from your client to ensure that it is positioned in the correct place (figure 6.24).

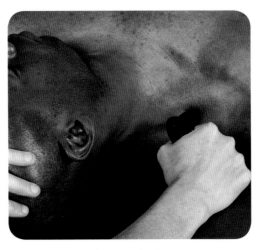

Figure 6.23   Using a massage tool to gently depress a trigger point in the upper, anterior fibres of the trapezius.

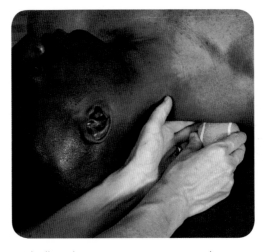

Figure 6.24   Using a ball to depress a trigger point in the posterior, upper fibres of the trapezius.

Step 2: With your thumb, tool or ball in place, maintain gentle pressure as you ask your client to slowly turn his or her head away from that side. For example, in the photographs shown in figures 6.23 and 6.24, the client would turn the head to the left. Lateral flexion of the head to that side also helps, but some clients find it difficult.

Advantage

- It is an effective way to deactivate trigger points in the upper fibres of the trapezius, as the muscle is relaxed when working with a client in the supine position.

Disadvantages

- It can be more difficult for some clients to actively perform lateral neck flexion.
- It can be more difficult to massage the area following the application of STR.
- It is not suitable for people with osteoporosis who should not receive deep pressure to specific points on the body.

Active STR for Upper Trapezius: Seated or Standing

Step 1: Sitting or standing, gently hook into the upper fibres of the trapezius using the end of a curved-handled umbrella (figure 6.25).

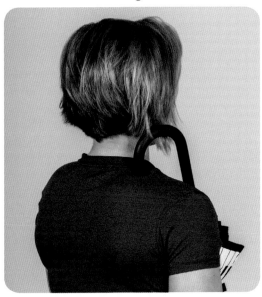

Figure 6.25   Using the curved handle of an umbrella to depress the upper fibres of the trapezius.

Step 2: Whilst maintaining the lock, either turn your head to the opposite side or laterally flex your head (figure 6.26). For example, when locking the fibres of the upper trapezius in the right shoulder, turn your head to the left or take your left ear toward your left shoulder.

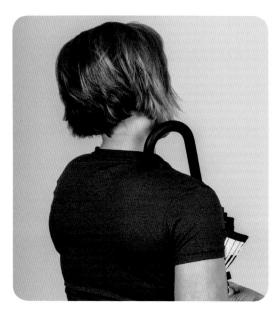

Figure 6.26   Laterally flexing the neck to bring about a stretch.

Whilst the upper fibres of the trapezius can be grasped in a pincer-type grip with the arm elevated instead of using an umbrella handle, STR in this position does not effectively stretch the tissues of the trapezius as pressure tends to come from the thumb that you are using to lock the fibres, and it is therefore more effective at treating the scalenes. Try this exercise for yourself: Sitting with your right arm elevated, use the finger and thumb of your left hand to gently pinch the upper fibres of your right trapezius. Maintaining your lock, turn your head to the left. Notice how you can feel more pressure from your thumb than you can from your forefinger—a stretch in the tissues on the front of your neck on the right side. Because your thumb is pressing into the very anterior aspect of trapezius, onto scalenes, it is a less effective method of active STR for the upper fibres of trapezius but a good way of stretching scalenes. Some people use a tennis ball to apply the lock, but it can be difficult to get into the right place to effectively lock the tissues of the upper fibres; although it can be helpful when locking the middle and lower fibres, should you want to apply STR there.

TIP   Practise active STR using one or both hands to depress the umbrella handle into the muscle in order to determine which is best. If you are applying STR to your right trapezius and depress the muscle using the umbrella in your left hand only, the advantage you have is that the muscle is relaxed but the disadvantage is that you are able to apply less pressure than when using both hands on the umbrella. When you use both hands to depress the upper fibres of the trapezius using the umbrella handle, you have more pressure and, additionally, the lower fibres of the trapezius contract as they depress the scapula. Activating the lower fibres in this way decreases tone in the upper fibres, which can be advantageous in bringing about a stretch and in deactivating trigger points.

Advantage
- Active STR to the upper fibres of the trapezius can be performed anywhere and with equipment as simple as an umbrella.

Disadvantage
- Where the upper fibres are hypertrophied it can be difficult to maintain a lock, as the umbrella hook slips off the muscle.

Active STR for Upper Trapezius: Supine

You can use active STR to treat the trigger point on the posterior of the upper fibres of the trapezius by resting on your back. Place a ball over the trigger point and turn your head to one side, as described in figure 6.24.

Advantage
- The muscle is relaxed, permitting easier access to the posterior portion of the upper fibres of the trapezius.

Disadvantages
- It can be difficult to access the anterior portion of the upper fibres of the trapezius.
- The weight of the shoulders on the ball can be uncomfortable for some people.
- It is not suitable for people with osteoporosis who should not receive deep pressure to specific points on the body.

Trigger Points in the Semispinalis Capitis

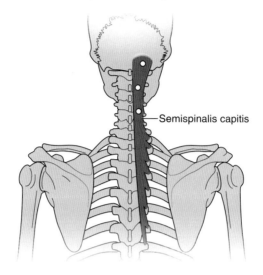

—Semispinalis capitis

Figure 6.27 Trigger points in the semispinalis capitis.

Trigger points can be found throughout the neck and thoracic extensor muscles. In their paper on trigger point injections for headache disorders, Robbins et al. (2014) provide guidelines for the reduction of trigger points in the semispinalis capitis and other neck extensors through injection. In addition, Fernandes-de-las-Peñas, Layton and Dommerholt (2015) have described the process for dry needling trigger points in the thoracic spine for the purposes of treating thoracic spine pain. For example, figure 6.27 shows some triggers in the spinalis muscle, located 1 to 2 centimetres (0.4-0.8 in.) lateral to the midline and referring pain to the temples, back of the head and base of the skull, radiating to the region of the posterior trapezius and up to the medial border of the scapula. They can be palpated either when the head is slightly flexed, tensioning the muscle slightly, or when the head is supported in a side-lying position and the muscles are relaxed. To locate the thoracic multifidus, place your finger immediately adjacent to the spinous processes of the spine, in the 'dip', and search for raised areas that refer pain when pressed. Trigger points in the longissimus thoracis muscle require palpation of the 'hump' of muscle running parallel to each side of the spine. Trigger points in the cervical extensors are perpetuated by postural stress or trauma to the head. Postures that might aggravate these triggers are slumped and forward-head postures, or where the head is held in an extended position for prolonged periods of time.

STR cannot easily be applied to trigger points in the posterior neck region, because to lock tissues here causes the neck to be pushed forward. Similarly, in the middle and lower regions of the thorax, the torso is pushed forward. In both cases this forward push causes the client to move away from you, making it difficult to secure the lock prior to a stretch. However, working in the upper portion of the torso, just inferior to the C7 vertebra does work and provides a nice stretch to the tissues of the posterior neck.

Active-Assisted STR for Erector Spinae: Seated

Step 1: With your client sitting, lock the tissues in the mid-thoracic area. In the photograph (figure 6.28), the therapist has chosen to use his knuckles.

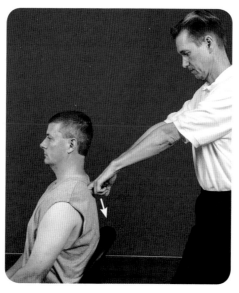

Figure 6.28   Locking the erector spinae tissues using the knuckles.

Step 2: Whilst maintaining your lock, ask your client to flex his or her neck (figure 6.29).

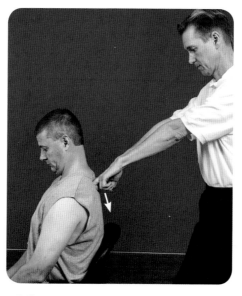

Figure 6.29   Active neck flexion brings about the stretch.

Step 3: Release and repeat, placing your lock slightly superior to the first one. Repeat as you work superiorly towards the neck. If you are performing STR correctly, your client will feel an increasing stretch as you move up the erector spinae.

Advantages

- Clients usually find this stretch to be comfortable.
- It can be performed with the client in a sitting position.

Disadvantages

- It is difficult to get a good lock on these tissues. As shown in figure 6.29, locking presses the client forward. It takes practice for the client to learn to remain upright, perhaps pressing back against your hands.
- It is easy to overuse your fingers or thumbs.

TIP Applying a small amount of massage medium and then working through a small towel or old T-shirt makes it easier to create a lock.

Trigger Points in the Scalenes

Trigger points in the scalenes (figure 6.30) refer pain to the chest, both the front and back of the shoulder, the medial border of the scapula, the front and back of the arm and the hand. They are most easily palpated using fingertip pressure as the client rests in the supine position. Although these muscles do not refer pain to the head, Florencio et al. (2015) found reduced pressure pain thresholds over trigger points in 30 women with migraine compared to 30 women without migraine, in not only those muscles known to refer pain to the head (suboccipitals, sternocleidomastoid and trapezius) but also in the scalenes and levator scapulae muscles. This finding lead the authors to recommend that neck musculature should be examined and treated in patients with headache.

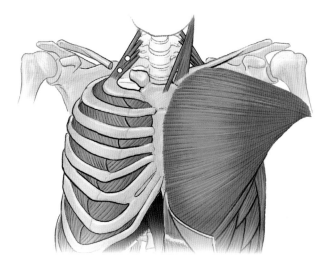

Figure 6.30 Trigger points in the scalenes.

Simons, Travell and Simons (1999) provide a long list of factors that activate and perpetuate trigger points in the scalene muscles. These factors include trauma, the actions of pulling and lifting as when hauling ropes, overuse of respiratory muscles, hard coughing, idiopathic scoliosis, playing some kinds of musical instruments and handling and riding horses.

Postulating that restriction of inspiration by respiratory muscles could impair function, Lee et al. (2016) carried out a study to examine the effect of stretching the scalenes, as they attach to the ribs and are therefore classes of muscles of respiration. They assigned 20 asymptomatic 20-year-old females into two groups, one used as a control group and one whose members carried out stretching of the scalene muscles. The slow vital capacity of each participant was measured before and after stretching using a digital spirometer. The stretching group followed a protocol in which they stretched anterior, middle and posterior scalene muscles, with the assistance of a practitioner, for a total of 15 minutes. Both inspiratory and expiratory volumes increased in the group who performed the stretching, leading the authors to conclude that stretching scalene muscles improved pulmonary function. It seems feasible that combining trigger point deactivation and stretching could have the same kind of benefit, and STR to the scalenes is one way to apply it.

Active-Assisted STR for Scalenes: Seated

Step 1: With your client sitting, gently lock the scalenes using your fingers (figure 6.31).

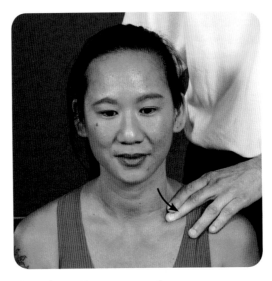

Figure 6.31   Gently locking the scalenes using a finger.

Step 2: Ask your client to rotate the head away from you until he or she feels a comfortable stretch in the tissues (figure 6.32).

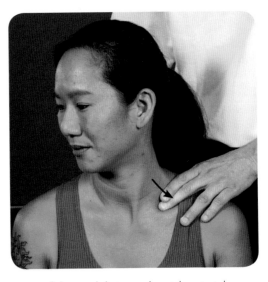

Figure 6.32   Active rotation of the neck brings about the stretch.

Step 3: Repeat the stretch three times on both the left and right sides.

Advantage

- When you work in this position, there is little danger that soft tissues of the neck will be overstretched, because the client is in charge of the stretch. Provided that the client is reminded to stretch only within a comfortable, pain-free range, it should always be a safe way to use STR to stretch this muscle.

Disadvantage

- It takes practice to fix the scalenes whilst avoiding the vascular structures of the neck.

Active-Assisted STR for Scalenes: Supine

Step 1: With your client in the supine position, gently palpate the scalenes and use your finger to create a gentle lock (figure 6.33).

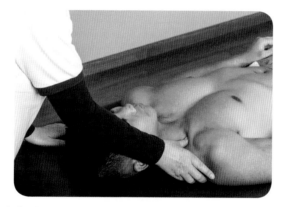

Figure 6.33 Gently locking the scalenes with a client in the supine position.

Step 2: Ask your client to turn the head away from you as you maintain your pressure (figure 6.34).

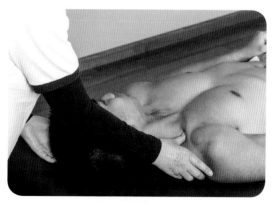

Figure 6.34 Active rotation of the neck brings about the stretch.

Advantages

- This is a particularly effective way of locating scalenes, as the neck muscles are relaxed.
- The technique lends itself to deactivation of trigger points that can be identified more easily in this position than when the client is seated.

Disadvantage

- As with application of active-assisted STR, when a client is seated, it takes practice to fix the scalenes whilst avoiding the vascular structures of the neck.

Active STR for Scalenes: Seated

Step 1: Sitting, standing or lying, use your right hand to gently palpate the scalenes on the left side of your neck. When certain you are on a muscle and not a vascular structure, apply gentle pressure using a finger (figure 6.35).

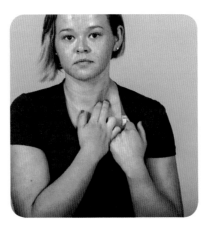

Figure 6.35 Gently locking the scalenes.

Step 2: Maintaining the gentle pressure, slowly turn your head to the right, stretching the soft tissues (figure 6.36).

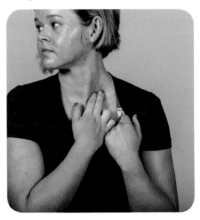

Figure 6.36 Stretching the scalenes whilst maintaining a gentle lock.

Step 3: Repeat the stretch on the other side, using your left hand to lock the right scalene muscles and then turning your head to the left.

Advantages

- It is a useful method of stretching the soft tissues of the anterior neck.
- It may be useful for the deactivation of trigger points in clients who feel uncomfortable when a therapist applies pressure to the neck.

Disadvantage

- Clients need to be taught not to press into blood vessels. However, it is unlikely that anyone would maintain pressure on a vessel as a pulse can easily be felt here.

Quick Questions

1. When a therapist applies passive STR to the rhomboids, why does the client need to have his or her arm positioned off the couch?
2. When applying active-assisted STR to the pectorals, how might you dissipate the pressure of your lock?
3. Why is active-assisted STR to the levator scapulae a relatively safe method of stretching neck tissues?
4. When applying active-assisted STR to the upper fibres of the trapezius, which bony structures should you be aware of?
5. When active-assisted STR is applied to the erector spinae, does the client flex or extend once you have locked the tissues?

Soft Tissue Release for the Lower Limbs

This chapter outlines how to apply soft tissue release to the lower limbs. You will find comparisons between applying passive, active-assisted and active STR to each of the major muscle groups of the lower body. Table 7.1 shows which versions of STR are presented in this chapter. The chapter also includes illustrations and information about trigger points found in each of the muscles.

Table 7.1   Types of STR Used on Muscles of the Lower Limbs

Muscle	Passive	Active-assisted	Active
Hamstrings	✓	✓	✓
Calf	✓	✓	✓
Foot	–	✓	✓
Quadriceps	–	✓	✓
Tibialis anterior	–	✓	–
Peroneals (Fibulari)	–	✓	–
Gluteals	✓	✓	✓
Iliotibial band (ITB)	–	✓	–
Iliacus	–	✓	–

■ *Passive STR:* Passive STR is excellent for treating the hamstrings, calf and gluteal muscles. Technically, passive STR can be applied to the foot, tibialis anterior, peroneals (fibulari), quadriceps, ITB and iliacus. However, doing so is either quite difficult or requires the therapist to adopt an awkward posture. Therefore, illustrations of passive STR to these muscles have not been included.

■ *Active-assisted STR:* As you can see from table 7.1, you are able to apply active-assisted STR to all muscles of the lower limbs. However, that does not mean that you should use this technique for all muscles. Practise the technique to discover the muscles for which you find active-assisted STR easiest to apply.

■ *Active STR:* It is possible to apply active STR to the hamstrings, calf, foot, quadriceps and gluteals by using a tennis ball. Active STR to the tibialis anterior, peroneals (fibulari) and iliacus is possible but difficult, so illustrations of this technique have not been included for these muscles.

The following sections provide detailed instructions for applying passive, active-assisted or active STR to many of the muscles of the lower limbs, including tips to help you along the way, and variations in treatment position where it is possible.

Trigger Points in the Hamstrings

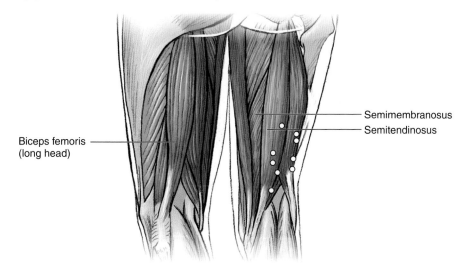

Semimembranosus
Semitendinosus

Biceps femoris
(long head)

Figure 7.1 Trigger points in the hamstrings.

Trigger points are found in the middle-to-lower portions of all three hamstring muscles—semimembranosus, semitendinosus and biceps femoris (see figure 7.1). Triggers here refer pain primarily to the back of the knee and proximal part of the posterior thigh and are perpetuated by activities such as sitting for prolonged periods of time with the knees flexed, as when driving or working at a desk, or when immobilized in bed or a wheelchair following injury or illness. Prolonged pressure to the back of the thigh is another perpetuating factor. You can palpate trigger points in this muscle group with your client in the prone, side-lying and even supine position, in each case with the knee flexed.

Using a group of 30 physically active males with tight hamstrings and at least one trigger point, Trampas et al. (2010) compared the effects of trigger point release combined with stretching with stretching alone and a control group. They took knee range of movement, stretch perception, pressure pain threshold and pain subjectivity measures (using the VAS scale) pre- and post- intervention. Non-painful cross-fibre friction massage was used over the trigger points in the trigger point plus stretch group. Both groups showed improvements in post-treatment measures compared to the control group who received no intervention; and the group who received trigger point massage as well as stretching showed a significant improvement in outcomes compared to the group who only received stretching.

TIP Pain radiating down the back of the thigh is not necessarily sciatica and can be an indication of trigger points in hamstrings.

Passive STR for Hamstrings: Prone

Step 1: With your client in the prone position, passively shorten these muscles by flexing the client's knee. Lock the muscle close to its origin at the ischium (figure 7.2) using your thumb or soft fist. Each time you lock the fibres in this stretch, direct your pressure towards the ischium rather than perpendicularly. When locking with a fist, make sure you keep the wrist in alignment; do not press through a flexed or extended wrist. If using your thumb to lock the tissues, take care to only press lightly as overuse may be damaging to your thumbs.

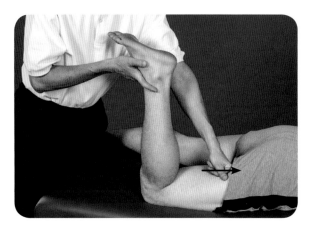

Figure 7.2 Locking the hamstrings as close to the ischium as possible.

TIP It's a good idea to explain to the client where the lock is going to be before beginning the treatment. Some clients may consider locking under the buttock in this way to be invasive. In figure 7.2, the therapist has chosen to place the first lock distal to the ischium, on the upper part of the thigh.

Step 2: Whilst maintaining your lock, gently stretch the muscle by extending the knee (figure 7.3). Many clients do not feel much stretch at this point.

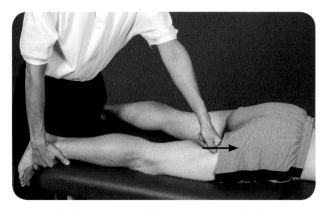

Figure 7.3 Stretching the hamstrings whilst maintaining a lock.

Step 3: Again with the knee passively flexed, choose a new, slightly more distal lock, perhaps in the midline of the thigh (figure 7.4).

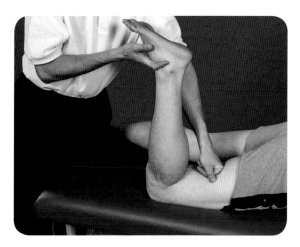

Figure 7.4 Creating a more distal lock on the hamstrings.

Step 4: Whilst maintaining your lock, stretch the tissues by passively extending the knee (figure 7.5).

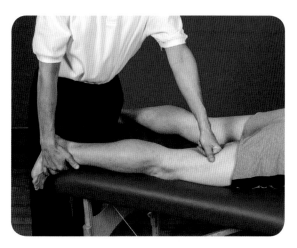

Figure 7.5 Stretching the hamstrings.

Step 5: Work down the length of the hamstrings from proximal to distal insertions, repeating this procedure. Avoid pressing into the popliteal space behind the knee. If you are performing the technique correctly, your client will experience an increasing sensation of stretch as you work towards the hamstring tendons. If your client does not feel the stretch, you will need to do active-assisted STR.

TIP You can use STR to help assess the pliability of the hamstring muscles. Notice the resistance you feel as you work from proximal to distal on these muscles. Can you sense which muscles are tightest—the biceps femoris (laterally) or the semimembranosus and semitendinosus (medially)?

If you wish to use STR to help deactivate trigger points, use your thumb to apply gentle pressure to a trigger, repeating the procedure over the trigger rather than to other parts of the muscle. Only when the trigger has dissipated should you move to another area. Following STR for trigger point release, instruct your client to perform hamstring stretches to maintain length in the muscle fibres.

Advantages

- Many clients report having tight hamstrings. This technique is helpful for assessing the pliability of hamstring muscles and identifying which muscles are tightest.
- Passive STR to the hamstrings may be incorporated into an overall massage treatment for the lower limbs with the client in the prone position.
- It is easy to use your thumb to gently lock trigger points you have located in the middle and lower portions of the muscles and to use passive STR to deactivate them.

Disadvantages

- The hamstrings are strong, powerful muscles that require a firm lock to fix the tissues. Using a fist to lock the tissues is one method of locking, but it is not as powerful as using a forearm (as in active-assisted STR).
- Elbows may be used to lock the tissues, but due to the length of the lever in this case, using the elbow makes passive flexion and extension of the knee difficult and may compromise your posture as you lean forward to lock the tissues.

Active-Assisted STR for Hamstrings: Prone

Step 1: Whilst your client is in a prone position, ask him or her to flex the knee. Using the side of your forearm or your elbow, lock the hamstrings close to the ischium (figure 7.6). Direct your pressure towards the buttock to take up some of the slack in soft tissues before the stretch.

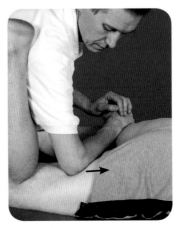

Figure 7.6 Locking the hamstrings close to the ischium using an elbow.

Step 2: Whilst maintaining your lock, ask your client to lower the leg back to the couch (figure 7.7). Release your lock.

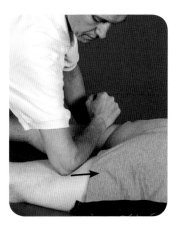

Figure 7.7 Stretching the hamstrings as the client lowers the leg to the couch.

Step 3: Choose a new lock, more distal to the first. Repeat the lock-and-stretch motion, working in lines down the posterior thigh from the ischium to the hamstring tendons. Avoid pressing into the popliteal space behind the knee.

TIP The knee does not need to be fully flexed at the start of the technique, or fully extended afterwards. Indeed, when working with a client with severe tightness on the posterior of the knee, full extension may not be desirable nor possible initially.

Advantages

- This method allows you to lock using the side of your forearm or your elbow and thus provides a stronger fix to soft tissues than when using a fist.
- Active-assisted STR to the hamstrings is particularly useful as part of the rehabilitation process after surgery to the knee or immobilization of the knee joint, by increasing knee range of motion and hamstring strength. Hamstrings contract concentrically each time the client actively flexes his or her knee; they contract eccentrically as the client lowers his or her knee, thus helping to maintain strength in these muscles.
- When the technique is used after knee replacement surgery, it may help increase both knee flexion and extension, because the client works within his or her pain-free range and is likely to increase range at the knee in a way that is safer than post-operative passive stretching.

Disadvantages

- Constant active flexion of the knee may cause the client's hamstrings to cramp.
- Leaning over to lock tissues could hurt your back so take care to guard your posture. Take a wide stance and ensure that your upper-body weight is supported by the client or treatment couch. With practice, this is easy.
- Use of the side of the forearm or elbow makes accessing trigger points in the medial aspect of the thigh tricky.

TIP Working on the leg closest to you (figure 7.8) is often easier than stretching across the body to the opposite leg. Using the right arm when treating the left leg (or left arm when treating the right leg) can also make application easier.

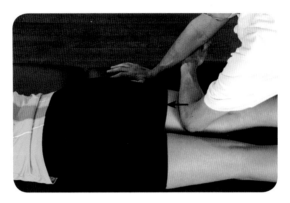

Figure 7.8 Applying STR to the leg closest to the therapist.

CLIENT TALK

Active-assisted STR has been great for treating a dancer who is flexible but nevertheless reports tightness in her muscles. The straight-leg raise test was not an appropriate method of testing hamstring tension in this client, who can easily position her chest on her thighs before and after treatment. Client feedback was therefore used to identify specific areas of tightness and work on and around those areas, sometimes with oil and sometimes without.

TIP Using the point of your elbow creates a more specific lock and can be a useful alternative to thumbs when using STR to deactivate trigger points which you have first identified with finger palpation (figure 7.9). However, it is more difficult to use the elbow in this way as you reach the distal end of the muscles, where a thumb lock is better.

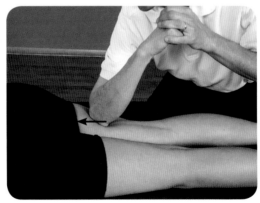

Figure 7.9 Using the point of the elbow to create a lock.

TIP An alternative position for treating trigger points in the hamstrings is to work with your client supine, his or her hip and knee flexed to 90 degrees. In this position you can grasp the distal point of the client's thigh above the knee, using your thumbs to press into the trigger points in this area. Maintaining pressure on the trigger, ask your client to slowly extend the knee until it is straight. Following trigger point release, your client is already in a suitable treatment position for passive hamstring stretch.

Active STR for Hamstrings: Supine

Step 1: Lie in the supine position, shorten the muscle by flexing your knee, and place a tennis ball over part of your hamstring muscles (figure 7.10).

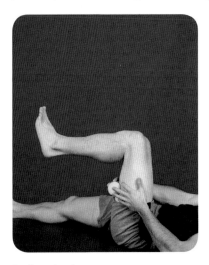

Figure 7.10 Applying a ball to the hamstrings.

Step 2: Whilst holding the tennis ball, gently extend your knee (figure 7.11).

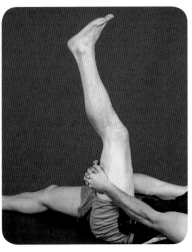

Figure 7.11 Stretching the hamstrings using a tennis ball.

Place your first lock (using the ball) near the ischium and gradually work down towards your knee with subsequent locks. Because the hamstrings are a large muscle group, you will need to work all over them to fully benefit from the stretches. Sometimes it is best to work systematically, perhaps starting with the biceps femoris on the lateral side of the thigh, proximal to distal (ischium to knee). When you feel you have worked this section enough, move your locks to a more medial position so that you are over the semimembranosus and the semitendinosus; continue to work this area in the same way. To use the technique to deactivate trigger points in hamstrings, palpate the muscle until you locate a trigger, place the ball over it, and repeat the STR on that same spot several times until the trigger dissipates.

Advantages

- It is easy to use active STR to deactivate trigger points in the hamstrings when resting supine.
- Elevating the leg helps blood and lymph drainage and could be a useful part of active recovery following exercise.

Disadvantage

- If you have large, strong hamstrings, it may be difficult to apply the necessary amount of pressure to lock the tissues with the ball in this position.

Active STR for Hamstrings: Seated

Step 1: With the knee bent as is usual when seated, place a ball beneath your thigh whilst sitting so that it is between you and the chair (figure 7.12).

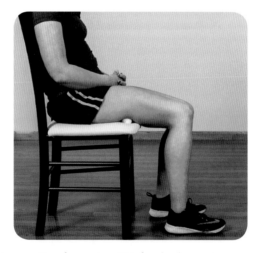

Figure 7.12   Starting position for active STR for the hamstrings.

Step 2: Extend your knee (figure 7.13).

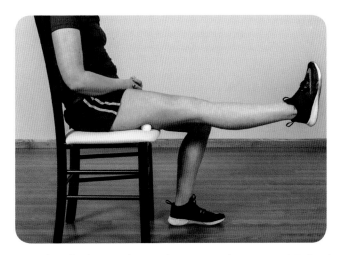

Figure 7.13 Extending the knee to bring about a stretch in active STR for the hamstrings.

Advantages

- Sitting STR is useful for treating hamstrings during the day if you have a desk job.
- Applying STR in a seated position is less effortful than when lying, as it does not require the ball to be held in place with the hands.
- It is relatively easy to use active STR to deactivate trigger points when sitting.

Disadvantage

- Active STR to the hamstrings when sitting places considerably more pressure on your hamstrings than when supine, and it could be painful.

Trigger Points in the Calf

Figure 7.14 shows trigger points in the medial and lateral portions of the gastrocnemius muscle. The medial triggers refer pain to the instep and medial aspect of the posterior knee primarily, radiating on the medial aspect of the calf, whilst the lateral triggers refer pain locally and to the lateral inferior knee region. These triggers are aggravated by forceful plantar flexion of the ankle as might occur when going *en pointe* in ballet or when walking up a steep hill. They are also perpetuated by compression of the calf, as when wearing tight socks or sitting with the legs outstretched, the calves resting on a footstool. Prolonged passive plantar flexion is also likely to aggravate triggers, as occurs when sleeping or wearing high heels.

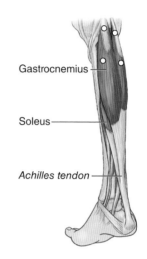

Figure 7.14 Trigger points in the calf.

Trigger points in the calf can be located with your client resting prone, their feet off the edge of the treatment couch (figure 7.15) or as they kneel on a chair, their feet off the edge of the chair, or with the client in the side-lying position.

Grieve, Barnett, et al. (2013) examined myofascial trigger point therapy for the triceps surae in 10 participants with calf pain. Baseline measurements were taken before and after each treatment; they were pressure pain threshold, presence of trigger points, ankle dorsiflexion range of movement, lower extremity functional scale and a verbal numerical rating scale. A therapist found trigger points in the gastrocnemius and soleus muscles using a thumb, then passively stretched the calf. Participants were also advised to self-treat their trigger points using a tennis ball or foam roller at least once a day, followed by active stretching of the calf. Thirteen active triggers had been identified at baseline across the 10 participants, and they were reduced to zero following intervention. However, the 31 latent trigger points which had been identified across the participants were only reduced to 30. Both ankle dorsiflexion for gastrocnemius and soleus improved post treatment, as did the pressure pain scores for all participants.

Grieve, Cranston, et al. (2013) also explored deactivation of latent triggers in the triceps surae of 22 recreational runners. Participants ran at least twice a week and had at least one latent trigger point in either the gastrocnemius or soleus. All had restricted ankle dorsiflexion. Trigger point release was performed with thumb pressure for 10 minutes followed by a 10-second stretch each of the gastrocnemius and soleus muscles. The control group received no intervention, but both groups had ankle dorsiflexion measures using a goniometer pre- and post-test. Ankle dorsiflexion increased in both groups but was greater in the intervention group. In the intervention group the increase was statistically significant compared to baseline measurements for both soleus and gastrocnemius, leading the authors to conclude that myofascial trigger point release provided an immediate improvement in ankle dorsiflexion.

TIP If a client complains of waking at night with a cramp in the calf, consider the presence of trigger points in the gastrocnemius.

Passive STR for the Calf Using Thumbs: Prone

Step 1: Position your client in prone with the feet off the end of the treatment couch (figure 7.15).

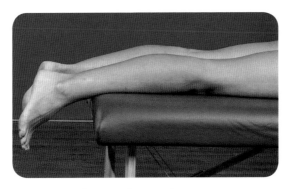

Figure 7.15   Positioning your client on the couch.

Step 2: Check for clips on the edge of the treatment couch that may press into the client's foot. Make sure the client can dorsiflex at the ankle. One way to do so is to gently push the ankle into dorsiflexion (figure 7.16).

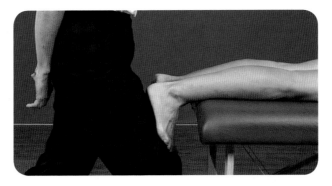

Figure 7.16   Passively dorsiflexing the ankle.

TIP Practise positioning your thigh on various aspects of your client's foot, either medially or laterally. Find the position that provides the client with the greatest stretch. When you apply this technique, you will need to provide passive dorsiflexion of the ankle to at least 90 degrees. Notice that to do so, you need to angle the client's foot so as to stretch the calf muscle, not simply press on the foot, thereby pushing the client up the treatment table.

Usually, it is best to shorten a muscle slightly before performing STR. The calf is an exception to this rule, because the foot and ankle naturally fall into plantar flexion, where the muscles are already in neutral, neither stretched nor contracted.

Step 3: Whilst standing at the end of the couch, lock the calf using reinforced thumbs, just distal to the knee joint, perhaps in the centre of the calf. Each time you lock the fibres in this stretch, direct your pressure towards the knee rather than perpendicularly (figure 7.17).

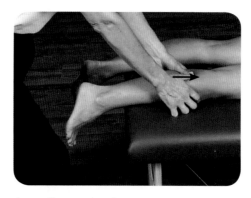

Figure 7.17   Locking the calf using thumbs.

To demonstrate passive STR to the calf, the therapist in figure 7.17 has used reinforced thumbs. This approach is useful in working through the following steps until you get the hang of passive STR. It is also a good way to treat trigger points in the upper part of the gastrocnemius (figure 7.14). However, it is essential for all therapists to protect their own limbs, and overuse of the thumbs should be avoided. Because they are plantar flexors, calf muscles are exceptionally strong, and it may be necessary to use a particularly firm lock when treating them. Although it may be tempting to press harder with your thumbs, you should avoid doing it.

Step 4: Whilst maintaining your lock, use your thigh to dorsiflex the client's ankle (figure 7.18).

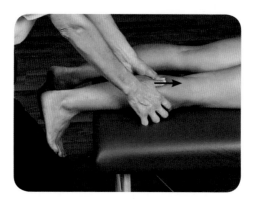

Figure 7.18   Stretching the calf passively by dorsiflexing the ankle using the thigh.

Step 5: Once you have dorsiflexed the ankle, release your lock, remove your thigh and move to a new locking position distal to your first lock (figure 7.19).

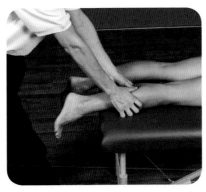

Figure 7.19 Locking tissues in the midline of the calf.

Step 6: Dorsiflex the ankle once again (figure 7.20).

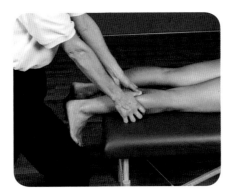

Figure 7.20 Passively dorsiflexing the ankle to bring about a stretch whilst maintaining a lock.

Step 7: Once you have dorsiflexed the ankle, release the lock and your thigh. Then, place a new, more distal lock (figure 7.21).

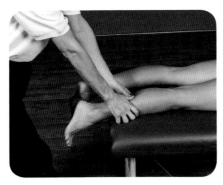

Figure 7.21 Creating a final, distal lock on the calf.

Step 8: Once again, passively dorsiflex the ankle (figure 7.22).

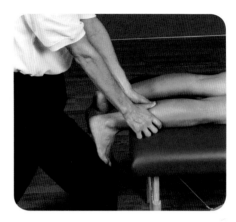

Figure 7.22   Passively stretching the calf whilst maintaining a distal lock.

Step 9: Work down the length of the muscle proximally to the junction of the muscle with its Achilles tendon. Repeat this action along the same line of the calf up to three times.

TIP   The gastrocnemius, the most superficial calf muscle, is a bipennate muscle; it has two bellies. Once you have performed STR down the centre of the muscle, move to the lateral or medial aspect of the calf, following the same steps. Working on the lateral and medial sides of the calf will help you to identify trigger points here. Notice that many clients have a palpable band of tension running down their lateral calf. Could this band be thickened fascia between the lateral and posterior compartments of the leg?

It does not matter whether you start STR in the centre of the calf or to the lateral or medial side. Usually, STR applied approximately three times to one group of muscle fibres is adequate to help stretch these fibres and increase range of motion at a joint.

Advantages

- Using the thigh to dorsiflex the client's ankle can provide a pleasant stretch in addition to that provided by the STR.
- This stretch may be incorporated into an overall massage treatment for the lower limbs with the client in the prone position.
- It is easy to palpate for trigger points in the calf and use STR to help deactivate them.

Disadvantages

- It is easy to overwork the thumbs.
- Clients with large, bulky muscles will not necessarily feel the stretch, because the lock will need to be firmer than the thumbs can safely apply.

Passive STR for the Calf Using Fists: Prone

The only difference between applying passive STR to the calf using fists instead of thumbs is in the method of locking. With your client in the prone position, follow steps 1 and 2 of passive STR to check that the ankle can be safely and comfortably dorsiflexed (figure 7.17).

Step 1: Instead of using thumbs, make a gentle fist to create the lock (figure 7.23).

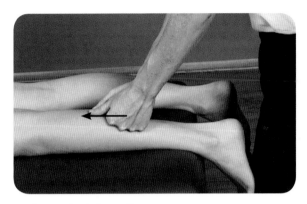

Figure 7.23 Using fists to lock the calf.

Step 2: Whilst maintaining your lock, gently dorsiflex the ankle (Figure 7.24).

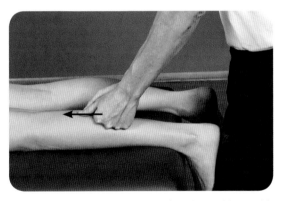

Figure 7.24 Using your thigh to passively dorsiflex the ankle and bring about a stretch whilst maintaining fist lock on the calf.

Advantage
- Using fists is a good alternative to save overuse of the therapist's thumbs.

Disadvantages
- It can be difficult to form a lock. Applying a massage medium and then working through a facecloth or small towel is helpful.
- This method cannot be used to treat trigger points.

Passive STR for the Calf Using Fists to Glide: Prone With Knee Extension

Step 1: Check that the ankle can be dorsiflexed (figure 7.17). Apply a small amount of massage medium such as oil or wax.

Step 2: As you dorsiflex the ankle, use your fist to apply pressure as you glide from the ankle to the top of the calf, reducing pressure when you reach the knee (figure 7.25).

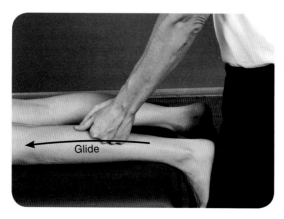

Figure 7.25   Applying gliding STR on the calf using fists.

Advantage
- It can be a soothing form of STR for clients with large, bulky muscles where you find it difficult to maintain a lock, or on those clients with tender calves for whom a specific lock is uncomfortable.

Disadvantages
- Although it is soothing to receive following deactivation using other methods, this method of STR cannot be used to deactivate trigger points.
- It requires a little practice to perform dorsiflexion whilst simultaneously gliding up the calf.

Passive STR for the Calf Using Forearms to Glide: Prone With Knee Flexion

Step 1: Rest your client's ankle on your thigh as they lie in the prone position, and place your hand on his or her toes (figure 7.26).

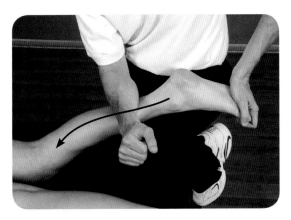

Figure 7.26 Placing the hands on the toes in preparation to glide up the calf.

Step 2: Using your forearm, glide from the ankle to the knee as you passively dorsiflex the ankle (figure 7.27).

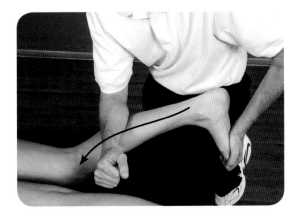

Figure 7.27 Passively dorsiflexing the ankle whilst gliding up the calf with the forearm.

Advantages
- Passive flexion of the knee helps relax the calf muscle.
- This method can also aid blood and lymph flow toward the knee.

Disadvantages
- Not all therapists find this treatment position comfortable.
- It can take practice to become proficient in passive dorsiflexion of the ankle with simultaneous gliding.

Active-Assisted STR for the Calf Using the Elbow: Prone

Step 1: With your client positioned as shown in figure 7.28, lock the calf muscle using your elbow. Place your first lock just inferior to the knee joint, taking care not to press into the popliteal space at the back of the knee. Notice that the muscle naturally falls into a neutral position with the client prone and therefore does not need to be actively shortened.

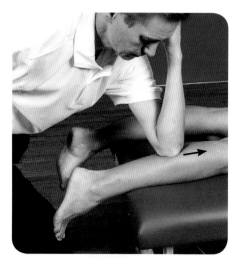

Figure 7.28 Gently locking the calf using the elbow.

Step 2: Whilst maintaining your lock, ask your client to pull up the toes, thus dorsiflexing the foot and ankle (figure 7.29). Once the client has done so, remove your lock and move to a new position.

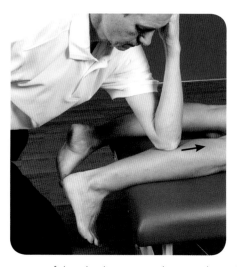

Figure 7.29 Active contraction of the tibialis anterior brings about the stretch.

Step 3: Repeat the action. Work down the calf towards the ankle, stopping when you reach the Achilles tendon. Repeat in lines from the proximal to the distal ends of the muscle.

Because constant dorsiflexion fatigues the tibialis anterior muscle, limit the time you spend on active-assisted STR to the calf.

TIP For an alternative to using your elbow, use your thumbs (figure 7.30). For a broader lock, use your forearm (figure 7.31).

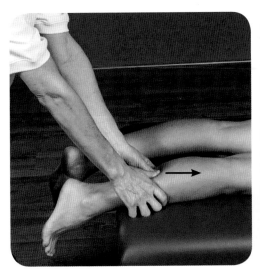

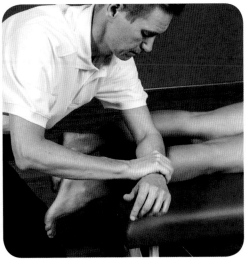

Figure 7.30 Using thumbs to lock the tissues at the start of active-assisted STR to the calf.

Figure 7.31 Using the forearm to lock the tissues at the start of active-assisted STR to the calf.

Whichever lock you use, make sure you transfer your weight to the client or to the couch: unsupported flexion of the trunk can cause backache.

Advantages
- This method enables you to apply a firm lock.
- Not having to stand at the foot of the treatment couch means that you can focus the lock in a variety of ways.
- The client is likely to dorsiflex to a greater extent than would be produced through passive STR to the calf and may therefore experience a greater stretch.
- Using the thumb or elbow is an effective method of deactivating trigger points.
- When used with permission from medical personnel, it is a great technique to incorporate as part of the rehabilitation process after Achilles tendon surgery. The client is unlikely to dorsiflex beyond his or her pain-free range and is therefore less likely to damage tissues through overstretching.

Disadvantages

- Constant dorsiflexion will eventually fatigue the tibialis anterior muscle.
- Leaning forward to lock using a forearm or elbow increases the possibility of injuring your lumbar spine. Make sure you transfer your weight to the client or to the couch.

Active-Assisted STR for the Calf Using Grip Lock: Prone

Step 1: Passively flex the client's knee, and grasp the calf (figure 7.32).

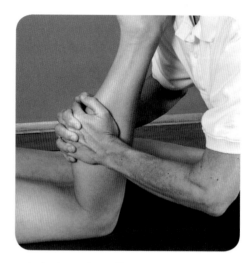

Figure 7.32   Using a grip lock on the calf.

Step 2: Whilst in this position, ask your client to plantar flex and dorsiflex the foot and ankle as you maintain the lock. Take care not to grip the muscle too hard.

Advantages

- The client does not need to position the feet off the edge of the treatment couch.
- Passive flexion of the knee facilitates slackening of the calf muscle, which permits a deeper lock and a different stretch sensation for the client.

Disadvantages

- It can be difficult to apply the lock along the length of the muscle. However, it may be possible to move a little either proximally or distally, depending on the shape and bulk of the calf.
- This method cannot be used to deactivate trigger points, as the lock is too broad.

Active STR for the Calf: Supine

Step 1: Resting with your legs outstretched, place your calf on a ball (figure 7.33). To shorten the calf, you would normally plantar flex. However, you will find that your ankle falls naturally into plantar flexion in this position.

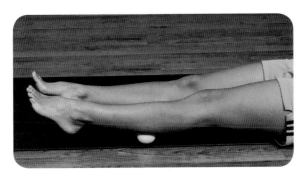

Figure 7.33   Positioning a ball to perform active STR for the calf.

Step 2: Gently dorsiflex your ankle (figure 7.34).

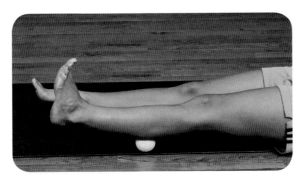

Figure 7.34   Dorsiflexing the ankle in active STR for the calf.

TIP   For a broader, less specific lock, an alternative is to place your leg on a cylinder, such as a can, and apply the stretch.

Advantages
- This technique is useful for overcoming cramping in an acute situation.
- It is a good technique for actively addressing trigger points in the posterior part of the calf.

Disadvantages
- Depending on how well-developed your muscles are, keeping your leg on the ball in this position can be tricky.
- This technique places considerable pressure on the calf muscles and may not be tolerable for all clients.

Trigger Points in the Foot

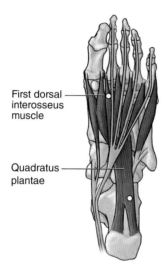

First dorsal
interosseus
muscle

Quadratus
plantae

Figure 7.35 Trigger points in the foot.

There are multiple trigger points in all of the muscle layers throughout the dorsal and plantar aspects of the foot. Figure 7.35 illustrates common triggers found in the deep, quadratus plantae muscle, which refers pain to the plantar aspect of the heel, and the first dorsal interosseous muscle, which refers pain locally on the dorsal and plantar aspects of the foot. Figures 7.36 and 7.38 show how these might be treated using a massage tool. These triggers can be perpetuated by trauma to the foot or by keeping the foot immobilized, as might be common following injury, or by tight fitting shoes. To palpate for any of the triggers in the feet, work slowly and in a systematic manner over the sole of the foot. Using the sit-and-reach and active knee extension tests pre- and post-treatment, researchers Patel, Vyas and Sheth (2016) examined the effect of self-treatment of trigger points in the sole of the foot in a group of 30 participants randomly assigned either a treatment or no-treatment group. All participants lacked 25 degrees of knee extension before the intervention, which was carried out over a period of four weeks. Participants were instructed to roll a tennis ball beneath the foot between the metatarsal heads and the heel, potentially releasing more than one trigger point, for a maximum of two minutes per foot, for one session only. Results showed that both the intervention and control group had significantly improved active knee extension scores, but there was no change in the sit-and-reach test scores. The authors concluded that a single session of self-release of the plantar fascia was beneficial in improving hamstring length but made no difference to lumbopelvic flexibility. They attributed the increase of hamstring flexibility in the control group to a training effect. That is, 'creep' of the soft tissues due to having taken three readings of the knee extension test.

Keep in mind that heel pain may derive from trigger points elsewhere, such as the calf, and some studies support the use of trigger point therapy to reduce heel pain. For example, Renan-Ordine (2011) carried out a randomised control trial of 60 participants with heel pain in which participants either self-released triggers in their calf muscles and also stretched the calf, or just stretched the calf. Outcomes were superior in the group who self-released triggers.

Active-Assisted STR for the Foot Using a Tool: Prone and Supine

Step 1: Position your client prone, with his or her feet off the couch and the ankle in a neutral position. Apply a gentle lock using a massage tool (figure 7.36).

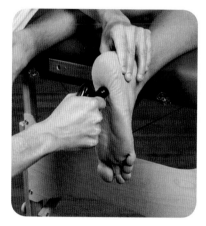

Figure 7.36 Using a massage tool to gently lock tissues on the sole of the foot when the client is in the prone position.

Step 2: Ask your client to pull up his or her toes, thus dorsiflexing the ankle and extending the toes (figure 7.37). Work over the sole of each foot for a few minutes only.

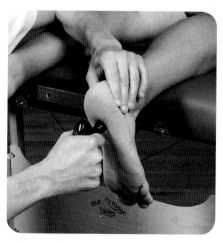

Figure 7.37 Actively dorsiflexing the ankle brings about the stretch.

You can also perform the technique with your client in the supine position (figure 7.38).

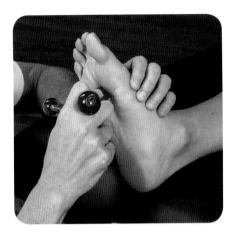

Figure 7.38   Applying active-assisted STR to the sole of the foot with the client in the supine position.

TIP   Whether using active-assisted STR in the prone or supine position, asking your client to extend the toes whilst also dorsiflexing the ankle increases this stretch. However, as most clients will not know what 'extend' means, you may need to ask them to 'pull up your toes even further' if they have not automatically done it.

Advantages

- Using a tool protects your thumbs.
- This technique may be incorporated into an overall massage treatment for the lower limbs with the client in the prone position.
- It is a useful way of addressing trigger points in the sole of the foot.

Disadvantages

- Not all clients like the sensation of the massage tool.
- Great care must be taken to avoid making too firm a lock.
- It can be difficult to get leverage here.

CLIENT TALK

A client trying to lose weight by walking to work started to experience foot pain when he changed from wearing training shoes to noncushioned flat-soled shoes. Having ruled out any serious pathology, the client received a foot and calf massage. He enjoyed the application of pressure to the soles of his feet, which was applied using a massage tool through a piece of tissue in order to get a secure lock.

Active STR for the Foot: Seated

Step 1: Whilst sitting down, place your foot on a tennis ball or spikey therapy ball with your ankle in neutral (figure 7.39). Notice that in this instance you do not need to shorten the soft tissues. To do so, you would need to flex your toes, and many people find this action causes cramping.

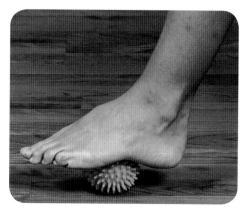

Figure 7.39   Resting the foot on a spikey ball to apply active STR.

Step 2: Gently extend your toes, dorsiflexing your ankle (figure 7.40).

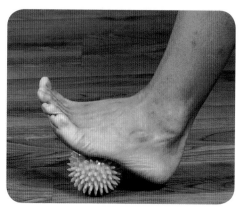

Figure 7.40   Dorsiflexing the ankle and extending the toes to bring about a stretch when using a ball for active STR of the sole of the foot.

Step 3: Work over the sole, moving the ball to discover which aspects of the fascia are tight and would benefit most from the stretch.

TIP   When working the plantar surface of the foot, it is also useful to treat the calf, because some of the calf muscles, such as flexor hallucis longus, extend down into the toes. Stretching the calf may help ease foot pain in some cases.

Advantages

- It is a useful way of addressing trigger points in the sole of the foot.
- Active STR for the sole of the foot is helpful for those clients who find active-assisted STR ticklish.
- Applying STR to the sole of the foot stimulates circulation and has been reported to help alleviate pain in people suffering from plantar fasciitis.
- This active stretch is a quick fix for clients who have been standing for long periods.
- It helps alleviate cramps in the foot muscles.
- It can help ease tension in the foot after prolonged walking or after running.
- The massage tool is easily portable.

Disadvantage

- Standing on the ball or overusing the technique can result in damage to the tissues.

CLIENT TALK

A client serving in the military police was experiencing plantar fasciitis in his right foot. He wanted to find a way to stimulate recovery because he had already had the condition in his other foot and found it debilitating. He was anxious that active-assisted STR might be painful and preferred to carry out his own STR, which he did successfully, using a golf ball instead of a spikey ball, over a period of weeks. Deep massage to the calf was used in helping alleviate tension in the connecting fascia, the aim of which was to take pressure off the calcaneus and perhaps also off the plantar fascia.

Trigger Points in the Quadriceps

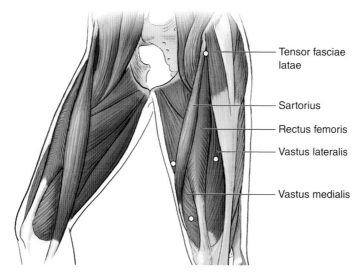

Tensor fasciae latae

Sartorius

Rectus femoris

Vastus lateralis

Vastus medialis

Figure 7.41 Trigger points in the quadriceps.

Four common trigger points are found in the quadriceps. The trigger point at the proximal attachment of the rectus femoris is close to the anterior superior iliac spine (figure 7.41) and refers pain into the knee. To identify the rectus femoris, palpate the area as you get your client to perform isometric knee extension in a manner that does not engage the hip. The rectus femoris will contract, and you will be able to palpate it for this trigger.

Two trigger points in the vastus medialis (figure 7.41) refer pain to the medial thigh and knee. To palpate for these trigger points, either stand facing the side of the couch with the client in the supine position and gently glide your fingers from the adductors through to the vastus medialis, or begin at the knee and palpate from the knee to the hip.

Trigger points exist in the proximal, distal and middle portions of the vastus lateralis, one of which is shown in figure 7.41. For more information on trigger points in this area, see the section on the iliotibial band (ITB).

There are trigger points in the vastus intermedialis (not shown in figure 7.41), and they refer pain over the anterolateral portion of the thigh.

The trigger points in the quadriceps are aggravated by trigger points in the hamstrings, and they may not resolve unless the hamstrings are first addressed. Tight hamstrings can prevent full knee extension, meaning that the muscle is unnecessarily strained during weight bearing. They are perpetuated by immobilization of the thigh, as is common following injury.

Espí-López et al. (2017) recruited 60 people with patellofemoral pain to compare the effectiveness of adding dry needling into trigger points to manual therapy and exercise. For 3 weeks, half the group received manual therapy and exercise and half the group received the same manual therapy, exercise plus dry needling into trigger points into the vastus medialis and vastus lateralis muscles. Outcome measures used were the Knee Injury and Osteoarthritis Outcome Score, the Knee Society Score, The International Knee Documentation Committee Subjective Knee Evaluation Form, and the numeric pain rating scale. Measures were taken at baseline, 15 days post-treatment and 3 months later. Both groups showed moderate-to-large improvements in all scores, no significant differences existed between the two groups, leading the authors to conclude that adding dry needling to trigger points to a manual therapy and exercise intervention did not result in improved outcomes for patients with knee pain and disability.

Active-Assisted STR for Quadriceps: Seated

Step 1: With your client sitting, lock the proximal portion of the quadriceps with the client's knee in active extension, directing your pressure towards the hip (figure 7.42).

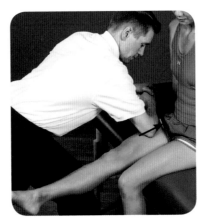

Figure 7.42 Locking the quadriceps using the soft side of the elbow.

Step 2: Maintain your lock as your client flexes the knee (figure 7.43).

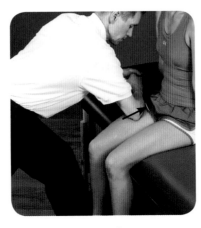

Figure 7.43 Active flexion of the knee as the therapist maintains the lock brings about a stretch in the quadriceps.

Step 3: Once the knee is flexed, release your lock and repeat, placing a new lock slightly more distal to the first. Work your way down the quadriceps from hip to knee.

Notice that the knee does not need to be fully flexed for the client to feel a stretch in the tissues. Practise locking the vastus lateralis and rectus femoris to locate areas of tension.

This stretch is particularly good for clients who have anterior knee pain aggravated by tight quadriceps. Work slowly and carefully as you approach the distal end of the quadriceps; it increases the stretch and thus places greater pressure on the patella.

TIP Although you can also perform this stretch using your left arm to lock the client's right quadriceps, both you and the client may find this position slightly invasive.

Advantages
- You will be able to achieve a strong, broad lock on these powerful muscles.
- You can use this method to deactivate trigger points in the thigh when they have been identified through palpation and the lock is created using the point of the elbow. In such cases, remember that your client will need to perform a quadriceps stretch following treatment to help maintain length in the muscle fibres.

Disadvantages
- Both you and the client may find this position slightly invasive.
- It is easy to compromise your posture. Therefore, to prevent unsupported forward flexion of the lumbar spine, use a wide stance.

Active STR for Quadriceps With a Tennis Ball

Step 1: Lie facedown on a mat, and position a tennis ball beneath your thigh with your knee in extension (figure 7.44).

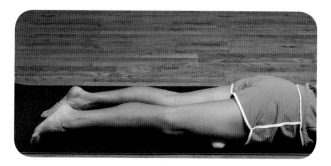

Figure 7.44 Positioning a ball at the start of active STR for the quadriceps.

Step 2: Flex your knee (figure 7.45).

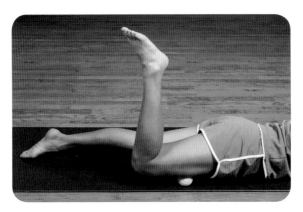

Figure 7.45   Active knee flexion brings about the stretch.

Practise positioning the ball against various parts of your thigh, and notice where you most feel the stretch. Position the ball first near your hip; with subsequent locks, work towards your knee. To help identify trigger points, use the ball and work systematically down the length of the muscles in this group. When you find a trigger, use STR to help deactivate it.

Advantages

- This method is useful if you find that a general stretching programme for your quadriceps is not targeting specific tissues. For example, by positioning the ball to the lateral side of your thigh, you are more likely to access the vastus lateralis.
- It is a good method for targeting trigger points in the rectus femoris and the middle portion of the thigh muscle.

Disadvantages

- Not everyone will feel comfortable in this treatment position.
- This technique may be uncomfortable for some people because the leg's entire weight is on the tennis ball. An alternative method is to use a massage tool to lock into your own thigh whilst sitting with your leg in extension.
- It can be difficult to treat trigger points in the vastus medialis using this method.

To apply STR actively to your quadriceps whilst sitting in a chair or on the edge of a massage couch, simply extend the knee and fix your quadriceps by pressing a ball into the tissues of your thigh. Maintain your lock as you gently flex your knee. Repeat this action several times on different parts of this muscle group. Accessing trigger points in the vastus medialis can be easier when seated.

Trigger Points in the Tibialis Anterior

A trigger point is found in the upper third of the muscle (figure 7.46) and refers pain to the dorsal aspect of the big toe and the front of the ankle. The point is easy to identify, just lateral to the ridge of the tibia. Trigger points in the tibialis anterior are likely activated by trauma to the ankle or foot.

Active-Assisted STR for Tibialis Anterior: Side Lying

For this stretch you will lock your client's tibialis anterior muscle. Sometimes you can position the client in supine. However, in figure 7.47, the therapist has positioned the client in side lying with her leg supported on a bolster in order to allow better access to the muscle. Notice that the therapist is supporting himself with his left hand on the treatment couch to avoid strain to his lower back.

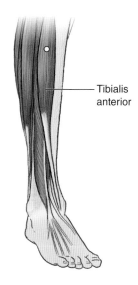

Tibialis anterior

Figure 7.46 Trigger points in the tibialis anterior.

Step 1: Locate the tibialis anterior by asking your client to pull up the toes. Whilst the client's ankle is in dorsiflexion, lock the muscle (figure 7.47). The tibialis anterior is a strap-like muscle, and the therapist in this photograph has chosen to lock it gently using his elbow, directing his pressure towards the knee.

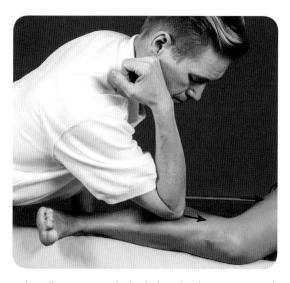

Figure 7.47 Using the elbow to gently lock the tibialis anterior with a client in the side-lying position.

Step 2: Whilst maintaining your lock, ask your client to point the toes (figure 7.48).

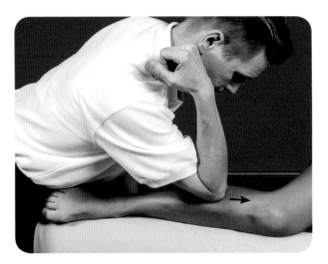

Figure 7.48   Active plantar flexion brings about a stretch in the tibialis anterior.

Step 3: Once the client has pointed the toes, release your lock and choose a new position, slightly more distal, for your second lock. With the ankle in dorsiflexion, lock in and repeat, working proximally to distally as long as the client feels the stretch and it is comfortable.

TIP   The tibialis anterior becomes tendinous fairly quickly, so it is not necessary to work all the way down the length of the muscle to the ankle; to do so may be uncomfortable for the client because this muscle lies over the tibia.

Advantages
- It is relatively difficult to apply passive or active STR to this muscle group, so active-assisted STR is a useful alternative.
- Once you feel confident locating the muscle with the client in this position, you may incorporate active-assisted STR into a massage routine with the client in supine.
- It is an effective technique for deactivating trigger points in the tibialis anterior.

Disadvantages
- This method may compromise your thumbs.
- If you use your elbow to lock the tissues, excessive pressure may damage tissues.

Active-Assisted STR for Tibialis Anterior: Gliding in Prone

Step 1: With your client in the prone position, apply a small amount of massage medium such as oil or wax to the front of the leg.

Step 2: Starting at the ankle, gently glide your fist along the length of the tibialis anterior muscle as your client actively dorsiflexes and plantrar flexes the ankle (figure 7.49).

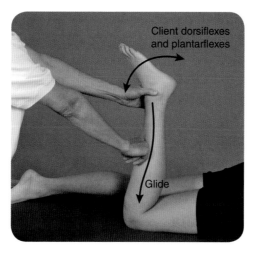

Figure 7.49   Using gliding STR on the tibialis anterior.

Advantage

- Treating the tibialis anterior in the prone position means that you can easily incorporate the technique into a regular massage routine.

Disadvantages

- You have very little leverage on the muscle in this position, so the stretch created is mild, which may not suit all clients.
- Gliding STR is not used to treat trigger points, as they require a specific lock to be held.

CLIENT TALK

Active-assisted STR to the tibialis anterior was combined with an oil treatment for a client with shin splints. In an attempt to give up smoking, the client had taken up running; thinking he could train hard and fast, he had been running every day for 3 weeks until his activity was limited by anterior shin pain. Stress fractures were ruled out, and STR was included in a gentle massage routine twice a week for 3 weeks. After a period of rest, the client was able to return to a gentler running programme.

Trigger Points in the Peroneals (Fibulari)

Trigger points in the peroneal (fibulari) muscles refer pain to the lateral malleolus, the anterolateral aspect of the ankle and sometimes to the heel (figure 7.50). You can easily locate them by palpating the lateral side of the leg with your client in a side-lying position. Take care when palpating the proximal end of the muscle, as the common peroneal nerve courses around the head of the fibula here and pressure to the nerve causes a tingling sensation.

Immobilisation of the ankle for any reason may perpetuate triggers, and clients with triggers may report frequent ankle sprains or feeling that the ankle is unstable. Other perpetuating factors include leg length discrepancy, flatfootedness, wearing high heels and prolonged plantar flexion.

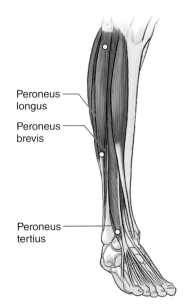

Peroneus longus

Peroneus brevis

Peroneus tertius

Figure 7.50 Trigger points in the peroneals (fibulari).

In a randomised controlled trial, Rossi et al. (2017) examined whether spinal and peripheral dry needling were any better than peripheral dry needling for people with a history of lateral ankle sprain. Twenty participants with a history of ankle sprain were randomly assigned one of two groups. One group received dry needling into trigger points in the multifidi and fibulari; the other group received dry needling to fibulari alone. Measurements were taken at baseline, immediately following the intervention and 6 or 7 days later. Measurements included the Foot and Ankle Disability Index, the Cumberland Ankle Instability Tool, unilateral strength, balance and hop test performance, and pain measured on the VAS scale. There was no significant difference between the groups at the end of the study, leading the authors to conclude that dry needling of multifidus in addition to dry needling of trigger points in fibularis muscles did not result in short-term improvements over and above dry needling trigger points in fibularis muscles alone.

Active-Assisted STR for Peroneals (Fibulari): Side Lying

Step 1: With your client in the side-lying position, ask him or her to evert the foot; demonstrate what you mean. Lock the muscle, which is now in a shortened position, directing your pressure towards the knee (figure 7.51). For demonstration purposes, the therapist in the photo has chosen to use reinforced thumbs to lock the muscle. Alternatively, you can use your elbow, using caution to prevent bruising the tissue against the fibula.

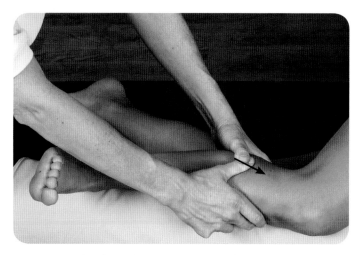

Figure 7.51 Using the thumbs to lock the peroneal (fibulari) muscles.

Step 2: Whilst maintaining your lock, ask the client to invert the foot. You may want to show the client how to do this motion first and, rather than use the term 'inversion,' ask him or her to 'turn the sole of the foot inwards' (figure 7.52).

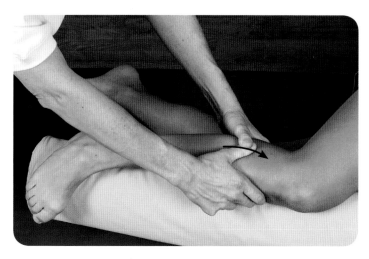

Figure 7.52 Active inversion of the ankle produces a stretch in the peroneals (fibulari) whilst the therapist maintains a gentle lock.

Step 3: Work in a single line down the muscle, from proximal to distal, as long as the client feels the stretch and remains comfortable.

TIP Clients with flatfoot have particularly tight peroneals and may benefit from stretching these muscles.

Advantage

- Active-assisted STR works best, because it is relatively more difficult to apply passive or active STR to this muscle group.

Disadvantages

- This technique may compromise your thumbs if overused.
- When using your elbow to lock the tissues, excess pressure can damage tissue.

Trigger Points in the Gluteals

Trigger points are found throughout all three gluteal muscles. Some are illustrated in figure 7.53. They are found in gluteus maximus, close to the lateral border of the sacrum; in gluteus medius, running inferior to the iliac crest and in the gluteus minimus muscle. The gluteus maximus trigger refers pain along the sacroiliac joint and into the base of the

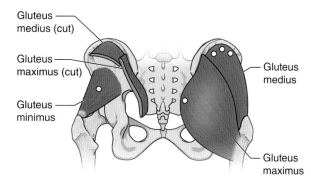

Gluteus medius (cut)

Gluteus maximus (cut)

Gluteus minimus

Gluteus medius

Gluteus maximus

Figure 7.53 Trigger points in the gluteals.

buttock on that side. It is easy to identify when your client is in a side-lying position. The gluteus maximus is associated with trigger points in the hamstrings and lumbar erector spinae, which are perpetuated by prolonged sitting and activities that require hip and spine extension such as repeated lifting of a heavy object.

The trigger points shown in gluteus medius refer pain to the sacrum, sacroiliac joint and ipsilateral (same-side) buttock. Palpate for these triggers with your client in either the side-lying or the prone position, sliding your fingers inferiorly off the iliac crest. Perhaps more than the other two gluteal muscles, trigger points in gluteus medius are perpetuated by gait abnormalities as might be caused by leg-length discrepancy or Morton's foot (second toe longer than the big toe). They are also aggravated by prolonged sitting and prolonged hip flexion.

Trigger points are found throughout the upper portion of gluteus minimus and refer pain to the buttock and lateral thigh and leg on that side. To palpate these trigger points, position your client supine, locate the tensor fasciae latae, and work your fingers posteriorly into the gluteus minimus. It is a deep muscle, and you are unlikely to be able to identify specific triggers easily but may be able to reproduce mild tenderness on applying pressure here. Trigger points in the gluteals are aggravated by prolonged immobility, either sitting or standing, and they are associated with trigger points in the quadratus lumborum muscle.

With all treatment, it is important to measure your effectiveness. Chapter 2 provided examples of various tests, such as the straight-leg raise test, which is one method of testing range of movement at the hip, notably length of the hip extensor muscles. Huguenin et al. (2005) examined the effect of dry needling trigger points in the gluteal muscles on the straight-leg raise test as well as internal rotation of the hip. They randomly assigned 59 male runners to a group that received dry needling to trigger points in the gluteal muscles or a group that received placebo needling to triggers. Triggers were reported in the majority of participants to be in the 'upper outer buttock quadrant' (p.87) and were pierced by the dry needle in one group, but in the placebo group the needle only touched the skin without piercing it. The straight-leg raise test and internal rotation of the hip were measured at baseline, immediately after intervention as well as 24 and 72 hours after intervention by taking digital photographs of the test positions. VAS scores were also recorded. There was no significant change in VAS scores or gluteal pain after running, but both groups showed significant improvement in reported hamstring tightness, hamstring pain and gluteal tightness after running. The authors commented that the results could indicate one of these three things: (1) The postulated restriction in range of movement measured by the straight-leg raise and internal rotation tests may not be associated with symptoms, (2) dry needling had no effect on muscle length in these muscles, or (3) the outcome measures used are not appropriate to measure change resulting from dry needling of trigger points.

Passive STR for Gluteals: Prone

Step 1: With your client in the prone position, grasp the ankle of the leg closest to you and flex the knee. Gently lock the tissues using your elbow, first or thumb. In figure 7.54, the therapist has chosen to use the elbow to lock fibres of gluteus medius.

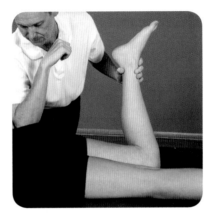

Figure 7.54   Gently locking the gluteals with an elbow.

Step 2: Maintaining your lock, rotate the femur by passively moving the ankle towards you or away from you, experimenting to determine where your client feels the stretch most (figure 7.55).

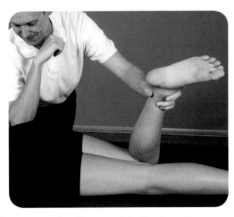

Figure 7.55   Passively rotating the femur whilst locking the tissues of the buttock brings about a stretch.

Advantages

- This method is an easy way to incorporate passive STR into a massage routine.
- It is also an excellent way to address trigger points in gluteals.

Disadvantages

- Pressing into the tissues too firmly using an elbow can cause damage to tissues.
- When using STR in this manner, it is difficult to access trigger points in gluteus minimus, as it lies towards the front of the hip.

Active-Assisted STR for Gluteals: Side Lying

Step 1: With your client in the side-lying position, the hip in neutral, use your forearm (close to the elbow) to lock the gluteals, directing your pressure towards the sacrum (figure 7.56).

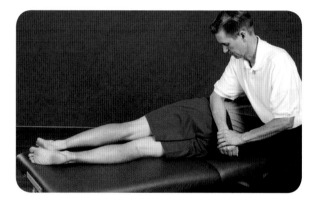

Figure 7.56   Locking the gluteals close to the sacrum with the hip in a neutral position.

Step 2: Whilst maintaining your lock, ask your client to flex the hip, perhaps by asking him or her to take the knee to the chest (figure 7.57).

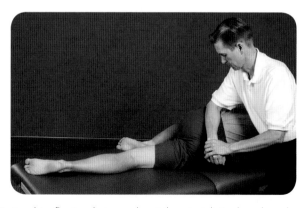

Figure 7.57   Active hip flexion brings about the stretch in the gluteals as the therapist maintains a passive lock on the tissues.

Step 3: Repeat this action for a few minutes, varying the position of your lock and working on the area that feels most beneficial for the client.

TIP It is quite challenging to apply active-assisted STR to the gluteals, and it takes practice to focus your lock in the correct spot on the muscles. With practice, however, you will discover a small area that, when locked, provides for the greatest degree of stretch.

Advantages
- Active-assisted STR to the gluteals in the side-lying position is helpful when working with a client who is unable to rest in the prone position.
- With experimentation is it possible to locate the fibres of the gluteus minimus, which are more difficult to access when using STR in the prone position. However, you may find that you need to lower your treatment couch to make working in this position more comfortable for you.
- With practice you will be able to identify triggers in the gluteus maximus and use STR in this position to deactivate them.

Disadvantage
- When you first begin, it is challenging to keep your client balanced in the side-lying position whilst you focus your lock in the correct spot on the muscles.

Active STR for Gluteals: Standing

Step 1: Stand with your back to a wall, and place a ball between your buttock on one side and the wall (figure 7.58).

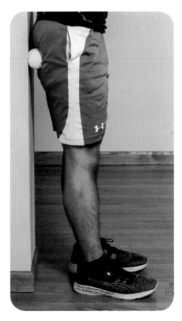

Figure 7.58 Positioning a ball at the start of active STR for the gluteals.

Step 2: Slowly flex your hip, bringing your knee to your chest (figure 7.59).

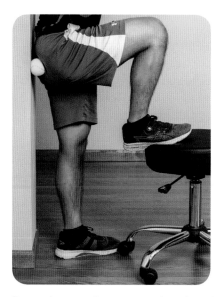

Figure 7.59 Active hip flexion brings about a stretch in the gluteal muscles.

TIP To stretch the gluteus medius and minimus, change your position so that your back is turned away from the wall or you are standing almost with the side of your body to the wall as you not only flex but adduct your hip. Notice how medial rotation of the hip can bring about a stretch in some parts of the gluteals once you have locked them using a ball.

Advantage

- Active STR to the gluteals is a good way to address trigger points in these muscles.

Disadvantage

- This technique requires you to stand on one leg as the hip is flexed, and this position can be a problem for people with poor balance.

Trigger Points in the Vastus Lateralis

The iliotibial band (ITB) is a thickening of the fascia covering the lateral side of the thigh and overlying the vastus lateralis (figure 7.60). Tender spots here are likely to be triggers in this muscle, and they refer pain throughout the side of the thigh from the hip to the knee. Palpate for these triggers with your client in the supine position, turned slightly away from you so that the lateral part of the thigh closest to you is raised off the couch a little. These trigger points are difficult to identify due to the thick fascial covering.

Pavkovich (2015) noted improvements in the Lower Extremity Functional Scale and Quadruple Visual Analogue Scale for four trigger points in the vastus lateralis, as well as those in the gluteus maximus, gluteus medius, piriformis and the greater trochanter area in a recreational walker with chronic lateral hip and thigh pain. Trigger points were treated with dry needling twice a week for 8 weeks. The patient reported a significant improvement in quality of life in terms of

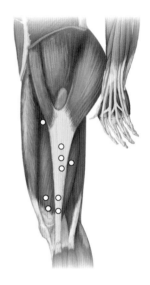

Figure 7.60 Trigger points in the vastus lateralis.

being able to sleep on the affected side, walk farther without pain and stand for extended periods. The author notes that strength in the lower limb improved and postulated that the improvement was a result of the participant having less pain and an improved gait posture.

Active-Assisted STR for Vastus Lateralis: Side Lying

Step 1: With your client in the side-lying position, check that he or she can flex the knee comfortably; if not, place a small towel or sponge between the client's knee and the edge of the couch. With the knee extended, direct your pressure towards the hip as you gently lock the tissues with soft fists (figure 7.61).

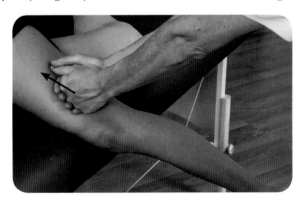

Figure 7.61 Gently locking the ITB with soft fists at the start of active-assisted STR.

Step 2: Maintain your lock as your client slowly flexes the knee (figure 7.62).

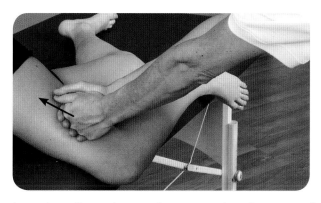

Figure 7.62   Active knee flexion brings about a stretch in the tissues of the ITB.

Step 3: Select a different lock position that is more proximal than your first, and repeat the procedure.

TIP   As for active-assisted gliding STR to the calf and tibialis anterior, you can modify this technique to the gliding form of STR too. Simply begin by applying a little massage medium, and place your lock just above the knee, gliding from the knee to the hip as your client actively flexes and extends the knee.

Advantage
- Active STR to the lateral thigh is a good way to address trigger points in the vastus medialis but only when fingers or thumbs are used to apply the lock.
- The technique can easily be modified into a gliding STR.

Disadvantage
- The side-lying position is not comfortable for all clients. Therefore, you must take care to protect the side of the knee resting against the couch.

Trigger Points in the Iliacus

A trigger point in the iliacus is located high in the muscle, just inferior to the iliac crest on the anterior of the ilium. It refers pain down the upper part of the anterior thigh. Palpate for it with your client in the side-lying position, hooking your fingers gently over the crest and pressing them towards you (figure 7.64). Prolonged hip flexion aggravates this trigger which is associated with triggers in the psoas and quadratus lumborum muscles. Ferguson (2014) provides examples of three case studies of clients with idiopathic scoliosis, describing how trigger points in muscles, including iliacus, affect and are affected by spine shape.

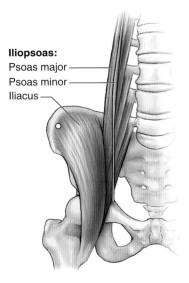

Iliopsoas:
Psoas major
Psoas minor
Iliacus

Figure 7.63 Trigger points in iliacus.

Oh et al. (2016) describe how an inflatable ball was used to deactivate triggers in a range of muscles, including the iliacus, in a group of elderly patients with chronic low-back pain. All participants had trigger points in the gluteus maximus, gluteus medius, iliopsoas and quadratus lumborum on at least one side that had persisted for more than 2 months. The iliopsoas was treated actively with the patient in the prone position; the hip on the affected side was abducted to around 45 degrees, and the knee was flexed to 90 degrees. Significant changes were found in VAS scores, pressure pain sensitivity and lumbar flexion.

Active-Assisted STR for Iliacus: Side Lying

This is an excellent stretch for clients with tight hip flexors. Show your client where you intend to place your hands, and be sure to get client approval before performing this stretch.

Step 1: With your client in the side-lying position and the hip flexed, lock into the iliacus on the anterior surface of the ilium (figure 7.64).

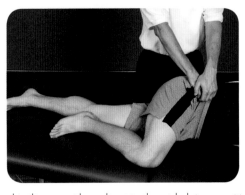

Figure 7.64 Locking the iliacus with a client in the side-lying position.

Step 2: Whilst maintaining your lock, ask your client to straighten the leg, which extends the hip (figure 7.65).

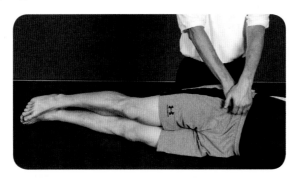

Figure 7.65 Active hip extension stretches the iliacus as the lock is maintained by the therapist.

The area to be worked is small, so the lock may be repeated in the same place or a centimetre to one side. Usually, performing the stretch three times this way will provide some relief from tension in the hip area.

If the client requires a greater degree of stretch, rather than pressing more firmly with your fingers, have your client extend his or her hip at the end of the movement. One way to explain this action is to ask the client to 'press into my fingers' when you get to the end of the movement.

TIP This area can be ticklish. An alternative is to ask the client to place his or her own hand on the area and then you press over it. Alternatively, dissipate your pressure by working through a facecloth folded into fourths.

Advantages

- Active-assisted STR works best because it is extremely difficult to apply STR actively or passively to this area.
- The abdominal contents fall away in side lying position, so having the client in this position is relatively safer than working with a client in supine.

Disadvantages

- This technique requires a fairly strong grip.
- The area may be ticklish.
- Some clients may find the technique invasive.

CLIENT TALK

An office cleaner came for treatment for lower-back pain. Tests revealed very tight hip flexors. The client frequently worked on her knees, in almost full hip flexion, causing shortening of her hip flexors and strain on her lumbar spine. After explaining the STR procedure using a miniature skeleton, STR was applied through her clothing twice a week over a period of 4 weeks to treat the iliacus. I also advised the client how to do active hip stretches.

Quick Questions

1. When performing STR to the hamstrings, which structure should you avoid locking into?

2. When performing passive STR to the calf, why do you use your thigh to dorsiflex the client's ankle?

3. Should you stand on a ball when performing active STR to the sole of your foot?

4. What sort of client might especially feel the stretch of STR to his or her peroneal muscles?

5. In which position do you treat iliacus—prone, supine or side lying?

Soft Tissue Release for the Upper Limbs

This chapter explains how to apply soft tissue release to the upper limbs. You will find comparisons between applying passive, active-assisted and active STR to each of the major muscle groups of the upper body. Notice, however, that not all three versions of STR can be applied to all muscle groups (see table 8.1).

Table 8.1 Types of STR Used on Muscles of the Upper Limbs

Muscle	Passive	Active-assisted	Active
Triceps	✓	✓	✓
Biceps brachii	✓	✓	✓
Shoulder adductors	✓	–	–
Infraspinatus	–	✓	–
Wrist and finger extensors	✓	✓	✓
Wrist and finger flexors	✓	✓	✓

- *Passive STR:* STR may be used passively on all muscles of the upper limbs with the exception of the infraspinatus, as passively rotating the entire upper limb medially whilst maintaining a lock is almost impossible.

- *Active-assisted STR:* Active-assisted STR works well on all of the muscles of the upper limb with the exception of the shoulder adductors, where it is difficult for the therapist to stand in a position to maintain a lock without getting in the way of the client's arm.

- *Active STR:* All the muscles of the upper limbs may be stretched using active STR, although this chapter has not shown active STR for the shoulder abductors or the infraspinatus.

The following sections provide detailed instructions for applying passive, active-assisted or active STR to many of the muscles of the upper limbs, including tips that may help you apply the techniques.

Trigger Points in the Triceps

Trigger points can be found throughout the triceps (see figure 8.1), including in the lateral and long heads of the muscle. The lateral trigger point refers pain to the posterior arm, sometimes radiating into the back of the forearm and fourth and fifth digits. The long head refers pain primarily to the shoulder and elbow, radiating along the posterior arm and forearm. Trigger points in this muscle are perpetuated through repeated or prolonged elbow extension. One way to palpate for these trigger points is with the client in the prone position, his or her shoulder abducted and elbow flexed, and the forearm resting over the edge of the couch. Explore the muscle with your fingertips, working consistently from the distal to the proximal ends.

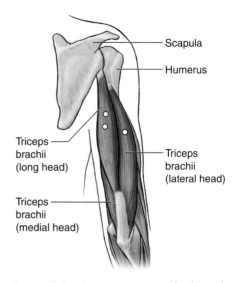

Figure 8.1 Trigger points in the lateral and long heads of the triceps.

Nielsen (1981) provided a good description of how trigger points were treated in the upper limb of a 59-year-old dentist with shoulder pain, beginning with the triceps. The subject was a keen racquetball player and had pain radiating down his arm into his hand. Nielsen examined each of the muscles of the shoulder, including teres major and latissimus dorsi. All muscles in which trigger points had been identified were treated by the spray-and-stretch technique in which cold spray is first applied to the muscle, which is subsequently stretched.

TIP If your client experiences a tingling sensation when you palpate for trigger points in triceps, this is the result of gentle pressure to the radial nerve. Tingling will resolve as soon as you reduce your pressure or palpate a different part of the muscle.

Passive STR for Triceps: Prone, Grip Lock

Step 1: Position your client in prone, and make sure he or she is able to flex at the elbow. Passively extend your client's elbow to shorten the muscle. Place your lock close to the origin, directing your pressure towards the shoulder (figure 8.2).

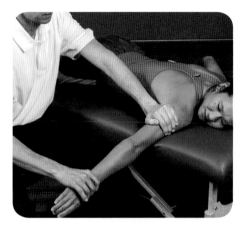

Figure 8.2 Using a broad grip to lock the triceps muscle.

Step 2: Whilst maintaining your lock, gently flex the elbow (figure 8.3).

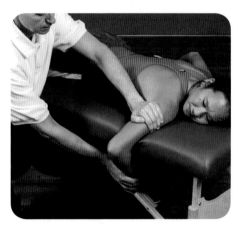

Figure 8.3 Passively stretching the triceps.

Step 3: Release your lock, extend the elbow and set a new fixing point more distal to the first. Repeat the action, working your way from the shoulder towards the distal end of the humerus. Your client should experience a greater stretch as you work towards the elbow.

Advantages

- This stretch is easy to apply, because the triceps do not need a very firm lock to stretch the tissues.
- By using a more specific lock, you can localize the stretch to particular tissues and especially to trigger points.
- Because you can use this technique with your client in the prone position, it is a relatively easy stretch to incorporate into a holistic massage.

Disadvantage

- It may be necessary to move your client to ensure his or her arm is fully supported on the treatment couch.

Active-Assisted STR for Triceps: Prone, Thumb Lock

Step 1: With your client positioned prone, create a lock on the triceps (figure 8.4).

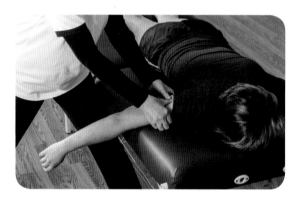

Figure 8.4   Locking the triceps.

Step 2: Ask your client to bend the elbow (figure 8.5).

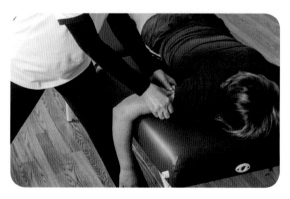

Figure 8.5   Active flexion of the elbow brings about the stretch in the triceps.

Advantage
- Active-assisted STR permits the therapist to lock specific points on the muscle, including trigger points, using a reinforced thumb if necessary.

Disadvantage
- Repeated elbow extension to bring the arm back to the start position can fatigue the muscle, and in this treatment position the elbow is extending against gravity.

TIP If using STR to deactivate trigger points in the triceps, remember to instruct the client to perform triceps stretches after the treatment. The elbow cannot flex fully when the arm is resting against the couch, which is the case with this treatment position.

Active STR for Triceps: Seated or Standing

Step 1: Extend your arm, and grip your triceps muscle (figure 8.6).

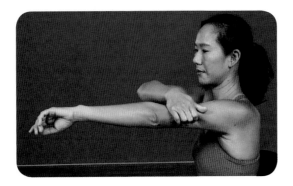

Figure 8.6 Gripping the triceps muscle.

Step 2: Whilst maintaining your grip, gently flex your elbow (figure 8.7).

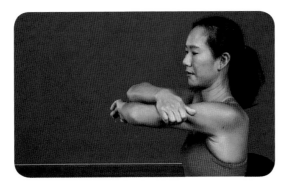

Figure 8.7 Active flexion of the elbow brings about the stretch in the triceps as a grip lock is maintained.

Some people do not feel the stretch in the triceps. However, most people will certainly feel it after activities involving prolonged or repeated elbow extension, such as when playing tennis or resting on the left hand whilst polishing with the right hand. Massage therapists who perform repetitive elbow extension when applying effleurage should practise active STR to the triceps between treating clients.

Advantages

- This stretch is easy to apply.
- Although applying a small lock actively can be tricky, a tennis ball placed between the triceps and a table can be utilised to target specific tissues or trigger points.

Disadvantage

- When you direct your pressure towards the shoulder, you take up slack in the tissues and get a better stretch. However, when working the triceps, it is difficult to direct your pressure towards the shoulder; as a result, applying the stretch actively is not as effective as when it is applied passively.

Trigger Points in the Biceps Brachii

Trigger points occur in both the long and short heads of the biceps brachii (see figure 8.8). They refer pain primarily to the front of the arm, proximally to the shoulder and distally to the elbow. They are perpetuated by repeated or prolonged use of the biceps as when flexing the elbow, lowering a weight against resistance or supinating the forearm, such as carrying heavy shopping bags, repeated loading or unloading of heavy items and fixing in screws using a manual screwdriver. Sometimes palpation for these points is easier when the elbow is passively flexed slightly. Begin at the distal end of the muscle, and work towards the shoulder, using your fingertips to explore the muscle fibres.

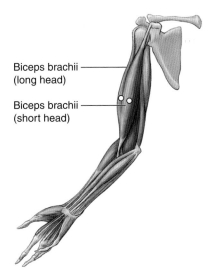

Biceps brachii (long head)

Biceps brachii (short head)

Figure 8.8 Trigger points in the biceps brachii.

Passive STR for Biceps Brachii: Supine

Step 1: With your client in supine and the elbow passively flexed, lock in gently to the biceps brachii, taking up slack in the skin as you direct your pressure towards the armpit (figure 8.9).

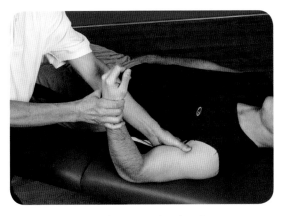

Figure 8.9 Locking the biceps brachii using the thumb.

Step 2: Gently extend the elbow whilst maintaining your lock (figure 8.10).

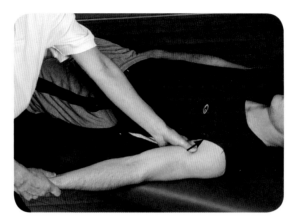

Figure 8.10 Passively extending the elbow whilst maintaining a lock brings about a stretch in the biceps brachii.

Step 3: Work from the proximal end of the muscle near the shoulder joint towards the elbow. Avoid pressure into the cubital fossa at the anterior of the elbow.

TIP When stretching out the biceps after using STR to deactivate trigger points, remember to pronate the forearm in addition to extending the elbow, because the biceps brachii is a forearm supinator.

Advantages

- This form of STR is easy to apply, because the biceps brachii does not usually require a firm lock.
- Because you can use this technique with your client in supine, it is a relatively easy stretch to incorporate into a holistic massage.

Disadvantage

- It may be difficult to fix large, bulky biceps due to their cylindrical shape.

Passive STR for Biceps Brachii: Supine, Gliding

Step 1: To modify passive STR to make it a gliding STR, begin by applying a small amount of massage medium to the biceps.

Step 2: Passively flex the elbow a little, and place a soft fist at the distal end of the arm. As you glide your fist from the elbow to the shoulder, simultaneously extend the elbow (figure 8.11).

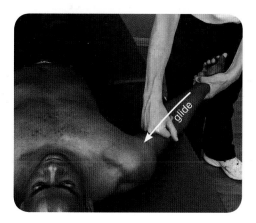

Figure 8.11   Passive gliding STR to the biceps brachii.

Advantage
- This massage is soothing to receive and can be helpful in stretching out tissues after locks have been placed to specific areas of the muscle.

Disadvantage
- Gliding STR cannot be used to deactivate specific trigger points.

Active-Assisted STR for Biceps Brachii: Supine

Step 1: With your client supine, ask him or her to flex the elbow. Then lock the tissues at the proximal end of the muscle (figure 8.12).

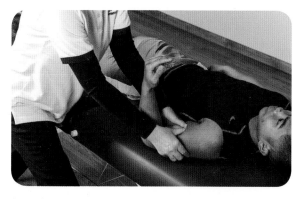

Figure 8.12   Locking the proximal end of the biceps brachii.

Step 2: Maintain your lock as your client actively extends the elbow (figure 8.13).

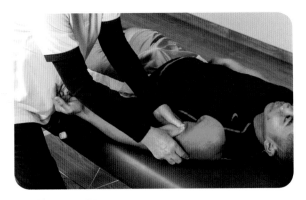

Figure 8.13   Active elbow extension brings about a stretch in the biceps brachii as the therapist maintains a lock on the muscle.

Step 3: Repeat the technique, each time using a new lock slightly more distal to the first.

Advantage

- Active-assisted STR facilitates locking of specific areas of the muscle, including trigger points, with greater pressure, should that be required.

Disadvantage

- Not all clients wish to be engaged with their treatment in this way when STR is incorporated into a massage, in which case passive STR to the biceps is more appropriate.

Active STR for Biceps Brachii: Seated or Standing

Step 1: With your arm in flexion, gently grip your biceps muscle (figure 8.14).

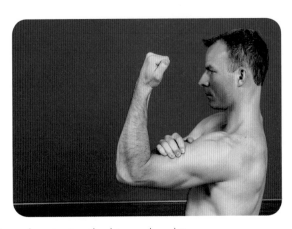

Figure 8.14   Actively gripping the biceps brachii.

Step 2: Gently extend your elbow whilst maintaining your grip (figure 8.15).

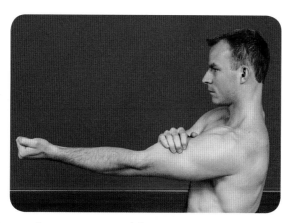

Figure 8.15   Active elbow extension whilst maintaining gripping the muscle brings about the stretch in the biceps brachii.

Applying STR to the biceps brachii feels good after any activity involving prolonged or repetitive elbow flexion, such as rowing, digging or carrying.

Advantage

- This stretch is easy to apply.

Disadvantages

- It is difficult to apply a small lock actively. Therefore, it is challenging to localize the stretch to specific tissues, including trigger points, unless a small ball is held over the point.
- It is difficult to direct your pressure towards the shoulder and take up slack in the tissues to get a better stretch.

Trigger Points in the Shoulder Adductors

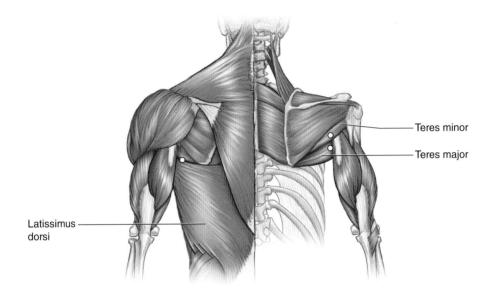

Teres minor

Teres major

Latissimus dorsi

Figure 8.16   Trigger points in teres major, latissimus dorsi, and teres minor.

The shoulder adductors include teres major, teres minor and latissimus dorsi posteriorly (see figure 8.16), all of which can develop trigger points, although some points are found more frequently than others. Trigger points in teres major and teres minor refer pain to the posterior deltoid whilst a trigger in the axillary portion of latissimus dorsi refers pain to the inferior angle of the scapula and down the entire upper limb posteriorly and anteriorly. Repeated adduction of the arm perpetuates trigger points in these muscles, which can be palpated with your client resting in either the prone or supine position, the arm passively abducted to around 90 degrees. If you are palpating the posterior axilla with your client supine, gently pinch the muscles between your finger and thumb; if you are working with your client prone, use your thumb to work along the lateral aspect of the scapula, identifying trigger points as you go.

Passive STR for Shoulder Adductors: Prone

Step 1: With your client resting in the prone position, his or her arm abducted to around 90 degrees, lock the tissues. The armpit can be sensitive to localized pressure, so the therapist pictured in figure 8.17 has chosen to lock the tissues using the palm and to apply gentle traction, which helps take up slack in the skin.

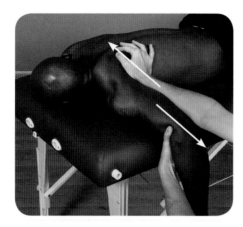

Figure 8.17 Locking the posterior shoulder adductors using the palm whilst applying gentle traction.

Step 2: Maintaining your lock, passively abduct the arm (figure 8.18). Notice how it feels for the client when you add gentle traction at the shoulder joint, but avoid tractioning the joint in clients who are hypermobile or who have a history of shoulder subluxation or dislocation.

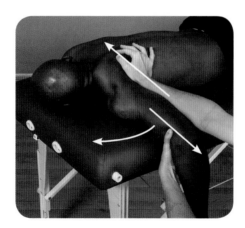

Figure 8.18 Passive abduction of the arm whilst maintaining a lock; traction brings about a stretch in the posterior shoulder adductors.

Advantages
- This stretch is easy to perform and relatively comfortable for most people to receive.
- You can use thumbs to lock specific trigger points and thus help deactivate them.

Disadvantage
- This area of the body is particularly sensitive, and specific locks using the thumb can be uncomfortable for some clients.

Passive STR for Shoulder Adductors: Side Lying

Step 1: With your client in a side-lying position, grasp the arm with one hand, passively abduct it to around 110 degrees and, using your forearm or elbow, gently lock the shoulder adductors.

Step 2: Maintaining your lock with your forearm or elbow, passively abduct the client's arm (figures 8.19 and 8.20).

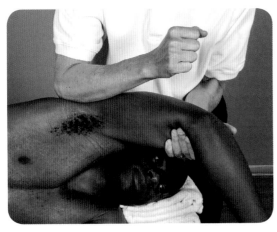

Figure 8.19 Passively stretching the adductors whilst maintaining a gentle lock using a forearm.

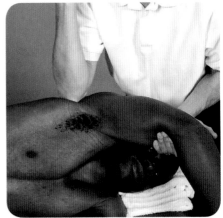

Figure 8.20 Passively stretching the adductors whilst maintaining a gentle lock using an elbow.

Trigger Points in the Infraspinatus

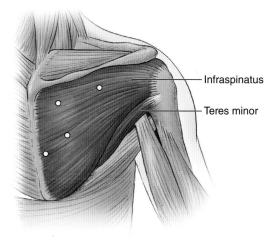

Figure 8.21 Trigger points in the infraspinatus.

Trigger points are found throughout this muscle (see figure 8.21). They refer pain to the front of the shoulder and medial border of the scapula, which can radiate down the anterolateral aspect of the arm. Palpate for these trigger points with your client in the prone position, his or her arms resting by the sides of the body. Trigger points here develop from sudden overload rather than overuse.

Hidalgo-Lozano et al. (2010) explored the relationship between trigger points and pressure pain hyperalgesia in 12 patients with unilateral shoulder impingement, 42 percent of whom had trigger points in the infraspinatus. Participants were asked to rate their pain on a numerical pain rating scale and to draw the location of their pain on a body map diagram. The pressure pain threshold over different trigger points was measured and compared to that of a control group of patients who did not have shoulder impingement. Significant differences were found between the two groups. For example, the patients had a variety of active and latent trigger points, whereas the control group only had latent trigger points and the patient group had a significantly lower pressure pain threshold. In the patient group, the intensity of pain correlated to the number of trigger points; the greater the number of trigger points, the greater the level of reported pain.

Active-Assisted STR for Infraspinatus: Prone

Step 1: Begin with your client resting prone, his or her arms by the sides of the body and externally rotated. The easiest way to achieve this position is to ask your client to turn the palms over so that they are resting on the treatment couch, as most clients rest with the dorsum of their hand on the couch when in the prone position. Apply your lock to the infraspinatus using your thumb (figure 8.22).

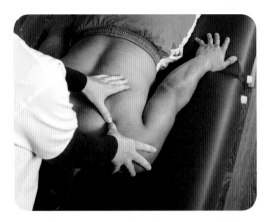

Figure 8.22 Locking the infraspinatus as the client rests with the arm externally rotated.

Step 2: Whilst maintaining your lock, ask your client to return to the position in which the back of the hand is against the couch (figure 8.23).

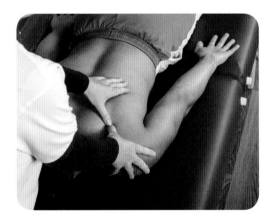

Figure 8.23 As the client internally rotates the arm whilst the therapist maintains a lock, the infraspinatus is stretched.

Advantage
- This method is effective for deactivating trigger points in the infraspinatus.

Disadvantage
- It can be difficult to maintain your lock on the infraspinatus as the client internally rotates the arm.

Trigger Points in the Wrist and Finger Extensors

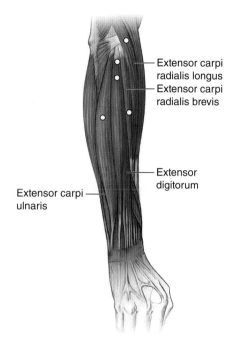

Extensor carpi
radialis longus

Extensor carpi
radialis brevis

Extensor
digitorum

Extensor carpi
ulnaris

Figure 8.24 Trigger points in the wrist and finger extensors.

Figure 8.24 illustrates trigger points found in the extensor carpi ulnaris, extensor carpi radialis longus, extensor carpi radialis brevis and extensor digitorum. The extensor cari ulnarus refers pain to the ulnar side of the wrist, the extensor carpi radialis longus refers pain to the lateral epicondyle and sometimes to the radial side of the dorsum of the hand, and the extensor carpi radialis brevis refers pain to the dorsum of the wrist and hand. The extensor digitorum refers pain to the dorsum of the middle and ring fingers as well as to the lateral epicondyle. Locate trigger points by gently rubbing your finger across the muscle fibres. You are likely to feel multiple taught bands of tissue. These trigger points are aggravated by prolonged gripping, as when carrying shopping bags. Triggers in the extensor carpi ulnaris are aggravated by holding the wrist in ulnar deviation, as might occur when using a computer mouse. Simons, Travell and Simons (1999) note that trigger points in the scalenes can result in satellite trigger points developing in the extensor carpi radialis and extensor carpi ulnaris. Trigger points in the extensor digitorum are perpetuated by repetitive movements, such as typing or playing the piano.

González-Iglesias et al. (2011) researched the effect of multi-modal treatment on nine rock climbers diagnosed with lateral epicondylitis. All completed a Patient-Rated Tennis Elbow Evaluation and their pain pressure thresholds were tested at baseline, after the third visit and 2 months later. Pressure to the extensor carpi radialis brevis replicated symptoms, so treatments included dry needling of trigger points to that muscle as well as manipulation of the cervical spine and wrist, mobilization of the elbow and taping. There was an improvement in all outcomes at both the final visit and the 2-month follow-up.

Passive STR for Wrist and Finger Extensors: Supine

Step 1: Gently extend your client's wrist. Lock into the bellies of the wrist and finger extensors on the lateral aspect of the forearm, directing your pressure toward the elbow (figure 8.25).

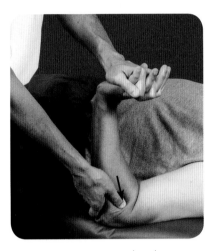

Figure 8.25   Locking the wrist extensors using a thumb.

Step 2: Whilst maintaining your lock, gently flex the wrist (figure 8.26). You can achieve a greater stretch by passively extending the elbow and flexing the fingers. It is difficult to do whilst maintaining a lock but can be achieved if you abduct your client's arm slightly when you extend the elbow so that the hand is off the treatment couch, thus facilitating flexion of the wrist and fingers. You will have to change the way you are holding the hand so that you can passively bring your clients fingers into a fist.

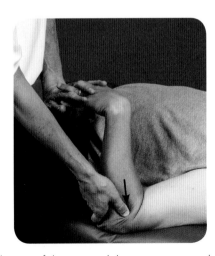

Figure 8.26   Passive flexion of the wrist whilst maintaining a lock brings about a stretch in the wrist extensors.

Step 3: Repeat the technique, each time selecting a lock more distal than the one previously used, as you work down the forearm from elbow to wrist.

TIP The muscles of the forearm are tightly bound in fascia, so to determine in which muscle you have located a trigger point, it is necessary to carry out active movement tests in order to identify a specific muscle. For example, the extensor carpi ulnaris extends the wrist and brings about ulnar deviation of the wrist, and asking your client to perform ulnar deviation once you have identified a trigger on the lateral side of the forearm is a relatively easy way to identify this muscle; the extensor carpi radialis extends the wrist and brings about radial deviation, so asking your client to perform radial deviation when palpating the medial side of the forearm is needed.

CLIENT TALK

Passive STR to the wrist and finger extensors was used in conjunction with a full upper-limb massage for a client recovering from lateral epicondylitis (tennis elbow) from playing tennis. The client was shown how to perform active STR in between treatment sessions, along with self-massage. She was advised not to apply active STR before playing tennis, because to do so might decrease her grip strength.

Advantages
- Because you can use this technique when your client is supine, this stretch is relatively easy to incorporate into a holistic massage.
- Little pressure is required to lock the tissues.
- It is easy to use this technique to help deactivate trigger points.

Disadvantages
- Getting the correct handhold so that you can flex and extend the wrist can be tricky when first learning the technique.
- It can be difficult to get leverage on the muscle bellies with your client in supine.

Passive STR for Wrist and Finger Extensors: Prone, Gliding

Step 1: Position your client prone with his or her shoulder abducted to around 90 degrees, the elbow flexed and the hand off the treatment couch. Check that you can passively flex the client's wrist. Apply a small amount of massage medium to the forearm.

Step 2: Passively extend the wrist. Beginning at the wrist, use your forearm or fist to slowly glide from the wrist to the elbow as you simultaneously flex the wrist (figure 8.27).

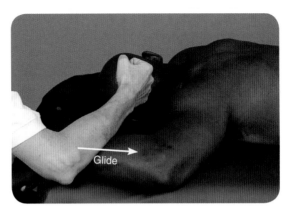

Figure 8.27   Gliding STR to the wrist and finger extensors.

Advantages
- It is a useful way of treating the wrist and finger extensors with a client in the prone position.
- Gliding STR is soothing following deactivation of trigger points.

Disadvantages
- Clients with shoulder problems may find abduction of the shoulder uncomfortable when performed in the prone position.
- Gliding STR cannot be used to deactivate trigger points.

Active-Assisted STR for Wrist and Finger Extensors: Supine

Step 1: Locate the bellies of the wrist and finger extensors by asking your client to extend his or her wrist. Lock the tissues using both thumbs, directing your pressure towards the elbow (figure 8.28).

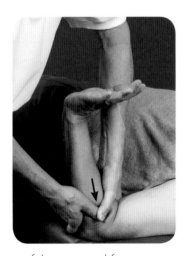

Figure 8.28   Locking the tissues of the wrist and finger extensors as the client actively extends the wrist.

Step 2: Whilst maintaining your lock, ask your client to flex the wrist (figure 8.29). Extending the elbow and flexing the fingers brings about a greater stretch.

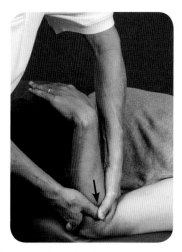

Figure 8.29   Active wrist flexion whilst the therapist maintains the lock brings about an even stretch in the wrist and finger extensors.

Step 3: Repeat the lock over the lateral aspect of the elbow where the muscle bellies are located.

TIP   This stretch is beneficial for the treatment of conditions such as lateral epicondylitis and for clients who perform repeated wrist extension, such as tennis players. However, the technique requires active wrist extension, so repeating the technique too many times within one treatment session may fatigue those muscles.

Advantages

- You are able to apply slightly more pressure using reinforced thumbs.
- Applying active-assisted STR is useful when working with clients who do not feel the stretch when it is performed passively.
- It is easy to use this technique to help deactivate trigger points.

Disadvantage

- It can be difficult to get leverage on the muscle bellies with your client in the supine position.

Active-Assisted STR for Wrist and Finger Extensors: Seated

Step 1: Position your client seated with the arm to be treated resting on a treatment couch and the hand off the couch. Check that the wrist can be flexed. Apply your lock at the proximal part of the muscle, using either your fist, forearm or thumbs, directing your pressure toward the elbow (figure 8.30).

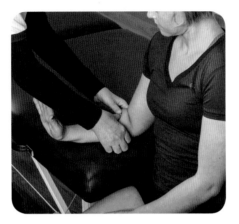

Figure 8.30 Applying a lock to the wrist and finger extensors with a client seated.

Step 2: Maintaining your lock, ask your client to flex the wrist (figure 8.31).

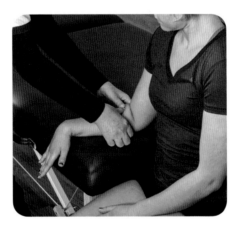

Figure 8.31 Active wrist flexion whilst the therapist maintains a lock brings about a stretch in the wrist and finger extensors.

TIP Look at the passive and active-assisted gliding techniques described in this chapter. Note that you could modify seated STR to make it gliding STR.

Advantages

- It is easy to get leverage on the wrist and finger extensors when treating them with your client seated.
- It is easy to use this technique to help deactivate trigger points.

Disadvantage

- STR used in this way is not incorporated into a massage routine.

Active-Assisted STR for Wrist and Finger Extensors: Gliding

Step 1: Position your client prone, with the shoulder abducted to around 90 degrees, the elbow flexed and the hand off the treatment couch. Check that your client can actively flex the wrist. Apply a small amount of massage medium to the forearm.

Step 2: Ask your client to extend his or her wrist. Beginning at the wrist, use your forearm or fist to slowly glide from the wrist to the elbow as your client flexes the wrist (figure 8.32).

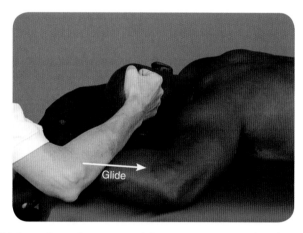

Figure 8.32   Gliding along the wrist and finger extensors as the client actively flexes the wrist.

Advantages

- It is a useful way of incorporating STR into a prone massage routine.
- Because the therapist has good leverage, it is a useful treatment position for addressing tension in the finger extensors.

Disadvantages

- Repeated active wrist extension against gravity can fatigue this muscle group.
- Gliding STR is not used to deactivate trigger points.

Active STR for Wrist and Finger Extensors: Seated or Standing

Step 1: Locate the bellies of your wrist and finger extensors. These muscles are on the lateral posterior side of your forearm. Gently lock into the tissues with your wrist in extension, directing pressure toward your elbow if possible (figure 8.33).

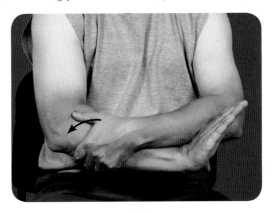

Figure 8.33 Actively locking the wrist and finger extensors.

Step 2: Whilst maintaining your lock, gently flex your wrist (figure 8.34).

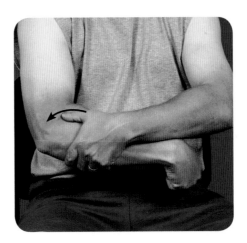

Figure 8.34 Maintaining a lock whilst flexing the wrist actively stretches the wrist and finger extensors.

Step 3: Work all over the extensors from proximal (near the elbow) to distal (near the wrist).

TIP Active STR is especially useful for people who spend a lot of time typing, anyone with tennis elbow and after activities involving gripping, such as carrying heavy bags, as it can easily be performed anywhere, at any time of day. It is great for massage therapists to use on their own forearms between treating clients.

Advantages
- It is a relatively easy stretch to apply.
- It can be used to deactivate trigger points.

Disadvantages
- It can be difficult to direct pressure both into the muscle and toward the elbow.
- It is easy to put excess pressure on the thumbs.

Active STR for Wrist and Finger Extensors: Gliding, Using a Roller

Step 1: Sit or stand with your forearm resting on a table, your palm turned upwards. Place a small roller beneath your forearm, beginning at the wrist, and apply gentle pressure using your other hand (figure 8.35).

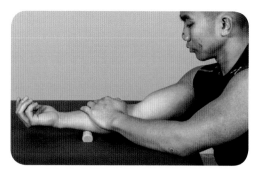

Figure 8.35   The start position for active STR to the wrist and finger extensors using a roller.

Step 2: As you roll your forearm over the roller from wrist to elbow, slowly flex your wrist (figure 8.36).

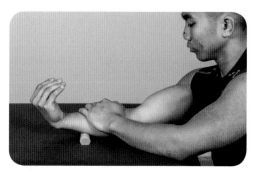

Figure 8.36   Flexion of the wrist whilst rolling from wrist to elbow brings about the stretch in the wrist and finger extensors.

TIP   To use the roller to help deactivate trigger points, simply rest the part of your forearm with the trigger point over the roller, then flex your wrist.

Advantages

- This stretch does not require any special or expensive equipment. Rollers are inexpensive, and you can use alternatives such as a can of food.
- You can use the roller to deactivate trigger points.
- It is an especially good method for addressing tension in the finger extensors.

Disadvantages

- It can take time to figure out which height works best for the treatment couch.
- It is often necessary to stand rather than to sit.

Trigger Points in the Wrist and Finger Flexors

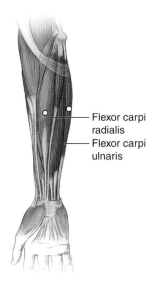

Flexor carpi
radialis

Flexor carpi
ulnaris

Figure 8.37 Trigger points in the wrist and finger flexors.

Figure 8.37 illustrates two of the trigger points found in the wrist and finger flexors, the flexor capri radialis and flexor carpi ulnaris, which refer pain to the middle and ulnar side of the wrist, respectively. Trigger points can be found in the flexor digitorum (not shown in the figure), and they refer pain to the dorsum of the middle, ring and little fingers. As with the wrist and finger extensor muscles, trigger points in the flexor groups are perpetuated by forced or prolonged gripping.

TIP To identify the muscle in which you have a trigger point, active wrist and finger movements are required. To identify the flexor carpi ulnaris, ask your client to bring about ulnar deviation; to identify the flexor carpi radialis, the client needs to bring about radial deviation; to identify the finger flexors, he or she needs to flex the fingers or bring about wrist flexion as you palpate the middle of the forearm.

Passive STR for Wrist and Finger Flexors: Supine

Step 1: Passively flex your client's wrist, and gently lock into the common flexor origin (figure 8.38). Holding the hand in such a way as to keep the fingers straight will facilitate this stretch.

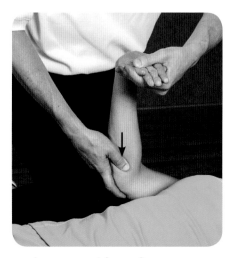

Figure 8.38   Locking into the wrist and finger flexors.

Step 2: Gently extend the client's wrist whilst maintaining your lock, preventing the fingers from flexing if possible (figure 8.39). Note that a great stretch is achieved if you also extend the elbow.

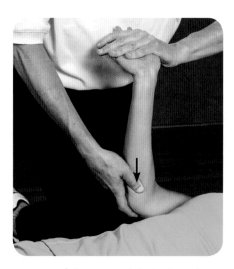

Figure 8.39   Passive extension of the wrist whilst locking the tissues brings about the stretch.

Step 3: Work down the forearm from proximal (elbow) to distal (wrist).

TIP You may find that it is better to work close to the origin of this muscle group, which quickly becomes tendinous in the forearm. Pressure into the anterior forearm is uncomfortable for some clients.

Advantages
- Because you can use this technique when your client is in the supine position, it is a relatively easy stretch to incorporate into a holistic massage.
- This technique can be used to deactivate trigger points.

Disadvantages
- Getting the correct handhold so that you can flex and extend the wrist can be tricky when first learning the technique.
- To fully stretch the wrist and finger flexors, it is best that the fingers as well as the wrist be extended (see figure 8.39), but it can be a difficult manoeuvre when you are using one hand.

Active-Assisted STR for Wrist and Finger Flexors: Supine

Step 1: Identify the muscles by asking the client to flex the wrist. Lock the tissues over the muscle bellies, directing your pressure towards the elbow (figure 8.40).

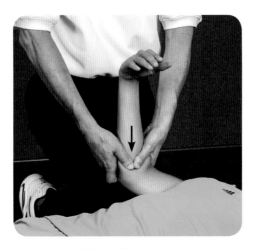

Figure 8.40   Locking the wrist and finger flexors.

Step 2: Whilst maintaining your lock, ask your client to extend the wrist (figure 8.41). Active extension of the elbow increases the stretch but can make it tricky to maintain your lock.

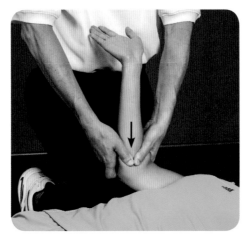

Figure 8.41   Active wrist extension brings about the stretch in the wrist and finger flexors.

Step 3: Repeat this lock-and-stretch, lock-and-stretch sequence over the muscle bellies.

Advantages

- You can apply slightly more pressure using reinforced thumbs.
- This technique is useful when working with clients who do not feel the stretch when it is performed passively.
- You can use the technique to deactivate trigger points.

Disadvantage

- It can be difficult to get leverage on the muscle bellies with your client in the supine position.

Active STR for Wrist and Finger Flexors: Seated or Standing

Step 1: Identify the bellies of your wrist and finger flexors. To do so, palpate your forearm on the anterior surface as you flex your wrist and fingers. You will discover the muscles on the middle and medial aspect of the forearm. With your wrist in flexion, gently lock into this area, gently pulling the tissues towards the elbow (figure 8.42).

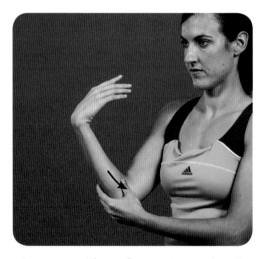

Figure 8.42 Locking the wrist and finger flexors close to the elbow.

Step 2: Whilst maintaining your lock, gently extend your wrist (figure 8.43).

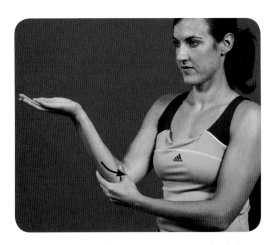

Figure 8.43   Active wrist extension whilst maintaining a lock brings about a stretch in the wrist and finger flexors.

Step 3: Work your way from the elbow to the wrist.

TIP   You may need to lessen your pressure as you work distally. The forearm becomes stringy with tendons and contains many neural and vascular structures that may be compressed on the anterior surface.

This stretch is great for people who type all day who are constantly flexing their fingers, and for drivers who, in gripping the steering wheel, are constantly working these muscles. It is also great for golfers and may alleviate the discomfort of golfer's elbow. Massage therapists who use their hands for applying petrissage should practise active STR to their wrist flexors between treating clients.

Advantages
- This stretch is relatively easy to apply.
- It is great for massage therapists to use on their own forearms between treating clients.

Disadvantage
- It is easy to place excess pressure on the thumb.

CLIENT TALK

I frequently apply STR to my own wrist flexors if I have had to carry heavy shopping bags or treatment couches. I also used it whilst writing this book when taking breaks from typing.

Quick Questions

1. When are you particularly likely to feel STR in the triceps?
2. In which position is the client when receiving passive STR to the triceps?
3. When performing active STR to the wrist extensors, do you start with your wrist in extension or flexion?
4. When performing active-assisted STR to the wrist flexors, do you lock in near the elbow or near the wrist?
5. Give examples of three clients who might benefit from STR to the wrist flexors.

PART IV

Soft Tissue Release Programmes

This part of the book tells you all about the client consultation process, gives examples of the kinds of initial questions you might want to ask and provides examples of the types of documentation some therapists use. Examples of commonly used assessments are provided in the sections on using a body map, measuring subjective sensations, postural assessment, range of motion and other special tests. Reading through the rationale behind the different consultation forms and comparing information from four very different case studies will give you a feel for how data are used to help design a treatment programme. Two of the case studies focus specifically on the use of STR in the treatment of trigger points.

Although therapists use specific consultation forms to ensure they meet the requirements of their regulatory bodies and insurance agencies, those provided here are useful examples. How do they compare to your own forms? Do you ask similar questions to those listed in the Initial Questions section? Do you use a body map, for example, or a visual analogue scale? Overall, this section is intended to help you identify how a treatment programme might be put together. It is *descriptive* rather than *prescriptive*. Use it to help you incorporate STR into your own treatment programmes, amending the various sections of your consultation process as necessary.

Creating a Soft Tissue Release Programme

Every therapist knows the importance of consulting with his or her client. The therapist needs to find out the reason the client has sought treatment, what the client expects from the treatment and, perhaps most important, whether any factors exist that may contraindicate possible treatment. Therapists use all sorts of forms to document information about the client. These forms include body maps, on which the therapist (or the client) highlights symptoms, and visual analogue scales (VAS), which are used to record the intensity of pain, stiffness or some other sensation. Most governing bodies and insurance agencies insist that therapists document treatments in detail. In addition, these agencies require that clients have consented to particular treatments and therapists have taken reasonable steps to ensure that the treatment is not contraindicated. These requirements are beneficial for everyone involved; they protect therapists, protect the client and help maintain a standard of professionalism. Although you may already be familiar with this sort of documentation, it is useful to review the rationale behind each of the consultation forms as well as compare these forms with ones you may already use. You may find this review especially helpful if you are a newly qualified therapist or practise bodywork other than massage.

It seems hardly necessary to mention the need for *etiquette-based medicine,* a term first coined by Kahn (2008) to describe the relationship between a clinician and his or her patient, as Kahn was referring to doctors treating patients in hospital and not to a clinician providing soft tissue therapy. However, where clients are being treated in a busy clinic, or who receive treatment from a multidisciplinary team, Kahn's comments are a touching reminder of some basic principles that therapists can overlook when they are trying to keep their appointments running on schedule and have commitments in the form of increased documentation (which is extremely common in the UK's National Health Service). Kahn thought teaching general good manners to medical students was required in order to tackle the problem of patient satisfaction, and suggested using a physician etiquette checklist. For example, for the first meeting with a patient in hospital, '1. Ask permission to enter the room; wait for an answer., 2. Introduce yourself, showing an ID badge., 3. Shake hands., 4. Sit down. Smile if appropriate., 5. Briefly explain your role on the team., 6. Ask the patient how she or he is feeling about being in the hospital.' (p. 1). It seems difficult to imagine a therapist not engaging with a patient (or client) this way, especially in a field where the environment is less medicalised and patient-centred care is highly regarded.

This chapter begins with some of the questions you might ask your client when he or she approaches you for the first treatment. As you read through these questions, you may want to tick off those you already ask and identify any that are new. Next, you can examine the body map chart and a visual analogue scale (VAS), two methods of recording information. In addition, you can also consider the value of carrying out a postural assessment and why range of motion (ROM) and other special tests might be used. Two case studies are provided, and you can examine how the information that was gathered affected the overall treatment programme. Also included are examples of the full documentation used for one of these case studies; the other is summarised. Finally, you can review two more case studies specific to the use of STR for the treatment of trigger points.

By the end of this chapter, you may have discovered some things you want to add to your own consultations. Perhaps you will simply feel reassured that the consultations you are currently carrying out are sufficient. Either way, with this knowledge you can start practising STR on yourself and your family, your friends and, of course, your clients.

Initial Questions

Your initial questions form part of your client consultation. The initial questions in figure 9.1 help you identify the reason for treatment and help provide clues as to the kind of STR that might be used, whether it is likely to be effective or whether it should be used at all. Some therapists like to use guided questions; others prefer to allow the client to tell his or her story in a semi-structured way whilst the therapist identifies and attributes the answers. All therapists aim to ask open-ended rather than yes-or-no questions; open-ended questions tend to elicit more information. It is also good practice to record answers using the client's own words as much as possible and to avoid prompting. It is sometimes tempting to ask, 'Where's the pain?' when a client may not have come to you with pain but with what he or she called 'stiffness' or 'something pulling'.

Asking questions is a skill, and it is perhaps the most important part of the consultation process. Effective questioning sets the scene for what is to follow. Clients need to feel at ease enough to tell you their stories. As a therapist, you need the confidence to identify and clarify salient comments whilst keeping the initial consultation within manageable time limits without making the client feel rushed. You may have already discovered how these initial questions determine the professional relationship you have with a client. When asked sensitively, these questions can help you gain rapport; when asked brusquely, hurriedly or in an offhanded manner, they can alienate a client.

INITIAL QUESTIONS

Client Name:_____ Date:_____

1. How may I help?

2. Where is the discomfort you described?

3. When did it start?

4. How was it caused?

5. Is it getting better, worse or staying the same?

6. Does anything make it worse?

7. Does anything make it better?

8. Have you had previous treatment for this complaint? Was it helpful?

9. Have you had this condition before?

10. Have you had any previous injuries to the same area?

11. Can you describe the type of discomfort you are feeling?

12. How does this condition affect your work and leisure?

13. Is there anything else you think I need to know?

Figure 9.1 Use these initial questions to identify the reason for treatment and to glean clues as to whether and how soft tissue release might be used.

From J. Johnson, *Soft Tissue and Trigger Point Release,* 2nd ed. (Champaign, IL: Human Kinetics, 2019).

In cases where you have to process a lot of information, it is often a good idea at the end of the initial question session to summarise your perception of the situation and state this summary to the client. For example, 'So just to be clear, you never had any leg problems before. A month ago you took up jogging and have since noticed a gradual increase in *achiness* in the front of your thighs. This achiness is uncomfortable when you stand up or when you sit on your heels but seems to go away within 24 hours if you rest. You copied some of the post-exercise stretches you found in a textbook for runners, and you admit to not doing them very often. Now when you try to stretch, the front of your thighs hurts even more.' This summary gives the client the opportunity to clarify any points. Perhaps he or she was not clear in describing what happened, or perhaps you misunderstood something. Sometimes hearing the story read back reminds the client of something he or she had forgotten all about. This situation is very common: A client says, 'Oh, I did get kicked in the thigh once, but that was ages ago. I'd forgotten all about that! I was playing football, and a boot went in my leg. It didn't bleed or anything; there was just this really big bruise, but it went away after a while. Could that have anything to do with it?'

One of the reasons therapists tend to ask so many questions and aim to work holistically is that, whilst a client may present with a hip problem, for example, an injury in one area can affect other parts of the body. A client might not be aware of the relevance of an old injury and so may either have forgotten about it or may discount it entirely, thinking it not worth mentioning. If a client comes with shoulder pain, for example, the client may not think to mention that he or she has recently recovered from a whiplash injury. Unless the client knows about anatomy, he or she may not be aware that some of the muscles of the neck also affect the shoulder.

Therapists of all disciplines who work in hospital and clinic environments often become highly skilled in asking these initial questions because they are working with strict time slots. They learn to identify which answers require further investigation and which ones are less important. Often, therapists also learn what kind of client they are dealing with, informing how to treat him or her. For example, someone who exercises regularly and intensely and with the tendency to acquire overuse injuries will respond differently to being told he or she needs to rest than will someone who has only just started an exercise programme and is keen to take as much advice as possible to avoid injury. In rare cases, it sometimes becomes apparent during this early part of the consultation that a client needs to be referred to another professional such as a doctor, podiatrist, radiologist or nurse. However you structure your consultation, by the end of the initial question session you should have formed an opinion as to why the client has come to see you, what and where the problem is and whether any contraindications exist to you carrying out further assessment.

TIP Making accurate, succinct summary statements is a skill in itself. If you want to boost your confidence in this area, try this method: Practise asking questions of a family member or friend, summarising what the person says. You need to find someone who has something that they might come to you with for therapy treatment. Practise asking questions and timing yourself to see how quickly you can identify the main problem, any contraindications and whether or not, after initial questioning, you may be able to help. Give yourself 20 minutes. Try again, giving yourself only 10 minutes. Can you identify any key questions from those you have asked that could have elicited the client's main issues in just 5 to 7 minutes had you asked them earlier in the interview?

In their paper titled 'Toward Patient-Centred Care: A Systematic Review of How to Ask Questions That Matter to Patients' Rosenzveig et al. (2014) say that patients' concerns must be elicited through direct questioning in order to establish the collaborative relationship between the patient and the clinician that forms the cornerstone to care. The authors carried out a systematic review of articles about the measurement of patient-reported outcomes that were designed to help inform patient-centred care and which did not include physical examination or performance testing. Measurements they found were about the patient's general health perception, stress, pain, fatigue, depression, anxiety and sleep. From their analysis of these measurements they created the visual analogue health state (VAHS) form, which contains clinically relevant, valid and reliable questions that one can use to structure conversations with patients. The VAHS contains seven questions, each ranked 0 (excellent) to 10 (poor); these questions are:

1. How would you rate your overall health?
2. How much distress are you experiencing?
3. How much pain are you experiencing?
4. How much fatigue are you experiencing?
5. How much depression are you experiencing?
6. How much anxiety are you experiencing?
7. How well are you sleeping?

Following are some of the questions you could use as part of your initial questioning session. They don't have to be asked in this order, and you may want to modify this list. As you can see, they are useful questions to ask when the client

CLIENT TALK

A client in considerable pain came to me for back massage after experiencing a very unusual accident. He was taking part in an exercise programme that involved galloping on a horse in a circus ring. Whilst trying to grip the horse with his legs, a safety harness attached around his waist pulled him off the horse. Whilst telling me this story, he stood up with great difficulty and, lifting the back of his shirt, he said, 'Look at this.' There were two very large bruises on either side of his lumbar spine. Clearly, this was an acute injury for which massage of any kind was contraindicated, and he was immediately referred.

comes to you with a specific injury or problem in a particular body part. However, many could be skipped if the client is coming to you for something simple such as a general maintenance massage. These questions are likely to be included in a consultation carried out by a massage therapist. Sports massage therapists, sports therapists, physiotherapists, osteopaths and chiropractors may choose to expand and adapt these questions. For this text, assume that the client is likely to need some form of massage, perhaps including STR.

1. *How may I help?*

Unfortunately, two of the most common opening questions are *Where's the pain?* and *So, what's the problem?* Neither of these questions is advisable, even when said invitingly, because although they are specific, they are also prompts. First, a client may not have any pain; he or she may have stiffness or tightness or a niggle. It's best to let the client report how he or she feels before using the same terminology yourself (say, 'A pulling feeling? Does it also pull when you look to the floor?'). Second, the client may not perceive his or her condition to be a problem at all. Many clients come for massage as part of a general maintenance programme. For example, runners may use it prophylactically to reduce the likelihood of developing problems associated with the iliotibial band; some weight trainers believe it helps reduce the likelihood of getting delayed-onset muscle soreness.

Choose an opening question that works for you. If it feels corny to ask, 'What may I do for you?' or too harsh to ask, 'So, why are you here?' then try being deliberately vague and ask, 'Anna mentioned it was your knee. Is that right?' This first question does not necessarily lead to a protracted explanation; it could equally take you to the heart of the issue. The client might tell you, 'The physiotherapist says I have a frozen shoulder. She wasn't sure but said it was ok to try massage if I thought that might help.'

2. *Where is the discomfort you described?*

The opening question should help determine the client's main complaint and the part of the body it affects, or any other reason for seeking treatment. If the client is describing a problem relating to a muscle, you need to determine whether the whole muscle or part of it is the problem. Some therapists, therefore, like to have a separate question that specifically asks, 'Where is the discomfort you described?' You might reword it for the situation, for example saying, 'Can you show me where it hurts?' or 'Do you feel the discomfort in the front of your knee or the back of it?' Soft tissue release can be used in stretching specific muscle fibres. Therefore, knowing that an old hamstring tear is in the biceps femoris, for example, is useful because it means you can later palpate and perhaps focus more on that hamstring with your treatment. Often, therapists will link this question to a body map (see figure 9.3) by writing *See chart*, or will make a small sketch if there is space on the consultation form. After subsequent treatments, you can refer back to this section to see whether the initial site of discomfort (if there was one) has moved.

3. When did it start?

This question helps you establish whether the problem had a gradual or a sudden onset. Is the client describing an acute condition, perhaps an injury he or she has just received such as a strained muscle, or did this condition happen some time ago? A calf muscle that was strained yesterday, for example, would be treated differently from a calf strain that occurred a week ago and is still causing problems. The more acute the strain, the less likely you are to apply STR. This question also helps identify overuse injuries. Overuse injuries such as tendinosis come on gradually and may be aggravated by repetitive activity. Often, a client cannot pinpoint when a condition started, yet his or her answers still provide clues as to whether the condition might be treated with STR. For example, a client may say, 'It comes on at work, when I've been on the computer for 4 or 5 hours.'

4. How was it caused?

An injury often has a known cause (e.g., the client tells you, 'I was running and then suddenly felt this sharp pain in my leg, and I couldn't run any more'), but with conditions such as sore muscles resulting from postural stress or overuse, the onset is so insidious that the client may not be able to identify the aggravating factor. You may hear statements such as 'Nothing caused it. It just hurts when I drive. It's worse when there's lots of traffic, and I have to change gears a lot. Then my arm starts hurting as well as my shoulder.'

5. Is it getting better, getting worse or staying the same?

Knowing how the condition behaves is especially useful within the context of STR. If a condition is getting worse, it could indicate that the client has an overuse condition that needs to be rested or that the client needs to be referred to another professional. Neither of these conditions should be treated with STR. On the other hand, if the client presents with tight hamstrings that seem to be getting tighter, it could indicate that STR would be beneficial.

6. Does anything make it worse?

Knowing what aggravates a condition is very helpful. Overuse injuries are aggravated by using the affected part. The answer to this question helps the therapist identify whether advising the client to rest and refrain from using that part of the body may be appropriate aftercare advice.

7. Does anything make it better?

Knowing alleviating factors is also useful. Clients who report that stretching helps ease pain, stiffness or discomfort may benefit from STR. Some therapists ask, 'Is there is anything you can do yourself that alleviates the problem?' Sometimes the client will make a direct statement, (e.g., 'No. It only stops if I stop cycling; when I rub it, it feels better') or will demonstrate a movement that he or she uses but cannot easily describe ('If I sit up straight like this it takes the pain away; sometimes I want to go like this. That seems to make it feel better for a bit.'). Muscle tension is often alleviated by stretching and changing position, so clients who report that these movements help may be more likely candidates for STR than those whose conditions may not be related to soft tissues.

8. Have you had previous treatment for this complaint? Was it helpful?

Sometimes you will not need to ask this question because the client will already tell you, 'Massage helps' or 'When I saw the osteopath it was fine for a while' or 'The woman in the gym fixed it last time.' You then can explore what the previous massage entailed, what the osteopath did or whether strengthening or stretching was used in the gym. If the client reports that he or she has had massage before and that it made the condition worse, you may be less likely to apply massage again. Conversely, the client may have had STR before and be able to tell you exactly where the therapist put his or her locks and how much it helped at the time.

9. Have you had this condition before?

If a client constantly experiences a particular condition, it may mean he or she needs more regular treatment, or it may suggest that an underlying condition needs addressing. Perhaps the client needs to alter his or her training routine. Surprisingly, clients sometimes repeat activities that bring about pain. Your client might say, 'I always get shin splints when I run on hard ground; I only get the neck pain when I drive for 4 hours without a break and forget to do my stretches.'

10. Have you had any previous injuries to the same area?

Although not always relevant, this question sometimes helps get to the bottom of long-standing problems. For example, a buildup of new scar tissue on top of an old injury that already has its own scar tissue may lead to an area of stiffness that requires a longer and more specific period of STR treatment.

11. Can you describe the type of discomfort you are feeling?

Some therapists like to ask this kind of question early in the interview, and sometimes the client describes his or her pain, stiffness or discomfort long before you ask about it (e.g., 'It just aches all the time when I'm writing'). Remember to document the client's own words. For example, if a client says, 'When I turn my head, it feels like something's getting squashed near my neck, here', this information is useful and quite different from your recording a statement that says, 'I have pain when I turn my head.' One of the best questions you can ask is 'How does it feel?' If you treat the client, you will probably want to check in with him or her to see if you have been effective. You can then ask, for example, 'Does it still feel like something's squashing when you turn your head?' Some therapists like to use a visual analogue scale (VAS; see figure 9.4) that measures the intensity of the client's feelings.

12. How does this condition affect your work and leisure?

This question provides all sorts of clues as to how quickly the client wants to recover if the STR is being used as part of rehabilitation (e.g., 'Once I can fully bend my knee, the doctor says I can go back to work'), how stressed he or she may be feeling (e.g., 'Everyone else is going. I feel like I'm letting the team down; If I could just do Thursday's match that would be great.') or whether the problem is limiting performance (e.g., 'I get worried that if I start to feel my hamstrings getting tight that I'm going to pull something. That happened last time, and I had to stop training for two weeks.'). Overall, this question may help identify how the client is likely to respond to treatment and what his or her treatment expectations are.

13. Is there anything else you think I need to know?

This is a vital ending question. You cannot possibly know everything about your clients. A client may respond with something very basic, such as 'Yes, I can only stay 30 minutes today because my child's minder is sick'; or he or she may say something that could have a direct impact on treatment but might not be picked up by the medical questionnaire, such as 'I want to try this again, but when I had treatment from that other practitioner, I felt a bit dizzy when I got up.'

The ways clients respond to your initial questions provide a wealth of information that is not necessarily the result of direct questioning. For example, their answers may reveal how they feel about therapy, medical professionals or their own body, and their responses often highlight yet more questions you need to ask. How a client answers opening questions provides hints as to how you might proceed with other parts of the consultation.

Client's Medical History

The client's medical history is of great importance; it not only helps you identify possible contributing factors to the problem for which the client hopes to be treated, it also helps you screen for contraindications to massage. Figure 9.2 provides a sample medical history form. Remember that contraindications to STR include easy bruising, thin skin and hypermobility syndrome. Other possible contraindications to massage or STR include recent physiological trauma, long-term steroid use, excessively high or low blood pressure, varicose veins, contagious skin disorders, heart problems, diabetes, osteoporosis and pulmonary oedema. In some of these situations, massage may be performed on some other parts of the body but not on the affected part. It is also important to remember that massage of any kind, including STR, is contraindicated in the first 12 weeks of pregnancy.

Using a Body Map

A body map (figure 9.3) is a useful, quick reference to which the therapist may refer before providing further treatment and for recording changes. It is simply an outline of the body, showing front, back and sometimes side views, onto which you record the area of your client's symptoms. It is helpful because you can see quickly whether tightness in the calf extends down the length and breadth of the muscle, or whether it is localized to a particular region, such as the Achilles. Some therapists use different types of shading to indicate differences in sensation. Darker shading might represent increased pain or increased stiffness, for example. Body maps may also be used to indicate areas where there were old injuries or local contraindications (such as athlete's foot, for example). When symptoms relating

MEDICAL HISTORY

Name:	Tel. No. (home) :	Tel. No. (work):
Address:	Mobile No.:	Date of birth:

Dr's name/tel no:

Address:

Occupation:	Weight:	Height:
Current medication:	Referred?	
Recent operations/illnesses:	Pregnancy:	

Circulation problems: (heart, pulmonary oedema, high/low blood pressure, poor circulation)	
Respiratory system: (asthma, bronchitis, hayfever)	
Skin disorders: (dermatitis, eczema, sensitivity, fungal infections)	
Muscular or skeletal problems: (fibromyalgia, previous fractures)	
Neurological problems: (sciatica, epilepsy, migraine)	
Urinary problems: (cystitis, thrush, kidney problems)	
Immune system: (prone to colds, reduced immune status)	
Gynaecological problems: (PMT, menopause, HRT, irregular periods)	
Hormonal problems: (diabetes)	
Digestive problems: (indigestion, constipation, IBS)	
Stress-related or psychological problems: (depression, anxiety, panic attacks, mood swings)	

INDEMNITY: I confirm to the best of my knowledge that I have not withheld any information relevant to my treatment and that I understand and accept full responsibility for the treatment that I am given. I also agree that I have given the correct information as detailed on this form, and shall inform the therapist should these circumstances change.

Client signature:_____

Therapist signature _____ Date _____

Figure 9.2 Every client should complete a medical history. From this form you will learn important information about the client, especially regarding contraindications for soft tissue release.

From J. Johnson, *Soft Tissue and Trigger Point Release*, 2nd ed. (Champaign, IL: Human Kinetics, 2019).

to several body parts need to be documented, some therapists like to indicate which is the main area, perhaps by using circled numbers 1, 2, 3 and so on, with 1 identifying the main area to be treated. As experienced therapists know, a body map does not always show the area of treatment, for the area where symptoms are being felt is not necessarily the area at fault.

Sometimes it is helpful to fill in the body map whilst showing it to the client and having the client confirm that you have marked the correct area. Some therapists decide to mark their body maps during the initial questioning phase of the consultation to get an overall picture of where problems are and where they have occurred in the past. This approach is especially helpful if there are many areas to be treated or a complex history of injury. Others prefer to complete the map either whilst palpating the client or after an initial massage treatment during which tissues are assessed. Recording information as the client gives it to you obviously documents what the client says and is regarded as part of a subjective assessment, whereas recording your own findings from palpation or massage is a form of objective assessment. It may not matter which method you use, as long as you remain consistent.

Another useful way to use the body map is to record the sites of trigger points. In this way you can refer back to the map during later consultations to determine whether your treatment has been effective at resolving any trigger points.

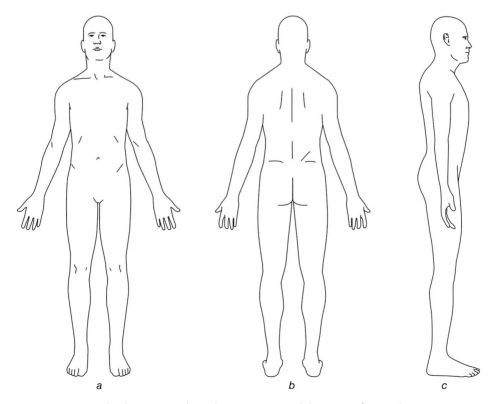

a   *b*   *c*

Figure 9.3   Use body maps such as this one to record the area of your client's symptoms.

From J. Johnson, *Soft Tissue and Trigger Point Release*, 2nd ed. (Champaign, IL: Human Kinetics, 2019).

TIP It is not always advisable to show your body map to the client after treatment if you are documenting your own objective findings. You have marked places all over the map, indicating where you found tissues to be particularly tight or areas of heat or increased sensitivity, and seeing so many markings could alarm some clients. They may away thinking that they have all sorts of things wrong with them, when in reality the map simply represents the subtle findings you have documented in a comprehensive manner.

Measuring Subjective Sensations

Figure 9.4 shows a visual analogue scale (VAS), which you may use to document subjective measures such as pain, stiffness, pulling sensation, or soreness. The scales are quick, easy and effective. Simply draw a line on a piece of paper. At the far left end write 'no pain' or 'no stiffness'; at the far right of the line, write the opposite—'worst pain ever' or 'maximum stiffness'. Show the line to your client, and ask him or her to mark it to indicate symptom intensity. After treatment, you may want to ask the client to mark the line again, using a fresh VAS. If the aim of your treatment was to reduce pain, for example, the client's new mark should be more to the left of the line. It is not always necessary to retest your clients in this way immediately after treatment. Sometimes it will be obvious that the treatment has helped by what the client says and does. Also, long-standing conditions do not necessarily resolve in just one treatment session. Several may be needed before you want to retest your client using a VAS. Gift (1989) makes the interesting point that not all patients can convert subjective feelings to a straight line. It is especially so when using VAS to ask about previous pain sensations, where a patient may not actually be able to remember the sensation.

The McGill Pain Questionnaire (Melzack, 1975) is one of the many methods for measuring pain. If you are working with a special population, such as children, the elderly or clients with whiplash, it would be worth exploring scales that have been used to measure sensations in that particular population. For example, Hawker et al. (2011) provides an overview of pain measurement systems used in rheumatology.

TIP Do not put numbers on your VAS. Clients remember numbers and may have a preference for a particular number. Or they may think that they should feel a lot less stiff, for example, and so mark a 3, remembering that their previous mark was a 6. If you were to test a client using a blank VAS, you may discover that whilst he or she did feel less stiff after treatment, this number was reduced to a 5 or even a 4 but not to a 3.

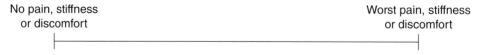

Figure 9.4   Visual analogue scale (VAS).

From J. Johnson, *Soft Tissue and Trigger Point Release*, 2nd ed. (Champaign, IL: Human Kinetics, 2019).

Postural Assessment

A quick postural assessment provides further information that may be relevant to the application of STR. Look for which of your client's muscles are short and tight and which are long and weak. Use STR to target the short, tight muscles, aiming to lengthen them, and avoid stretching the muscles that are already too long. Generally, when chest muscles (e.g., pectoralis major) are tight, muscles of the thoracic spine (e.g., middle fibres of trapezius) are longer and weaker; when abdominals are weak, muscles of the lumbar spine (e.g., erector spinae) and hip flexors (e.g., psoas muscles) are tight. For more information on postural assessment, look at *Postural Assessment* by Jane Johnson and *Muscles: Testing and Function with Posture and Pain* by Florence Peterson Kendall, Elizabeth Kendall McCreary, Patricia Geise Provance, Mary McIntyre Rodgers and William Anthony Romani.

Range of Motion and Other Special Tests

If STR is being used to increase range of motion (ROM), then it may be useful to complete a chart highlighting the ROM of the joints relating to the area and muscles being treated. For example, if a client is being treated for tight or painful shoulders, knowing the ROM at the glenohumeral joint would be useful to assess limitations and to gauge the effectiveness of treatment. Other special tests include the straight-leg raise for hamstring length (figure 2.2), the prone knee bend test for the length of the quadriceps (figure 2.3), the sit-and-reach-test for hamstring and spine length (figure 2.4), the Thomas test (for hip flexor length), the Ober test (for tightness in the iliotibial band) and differentiation tests for tightness between the soleus and the gastrocnemius.

Programme for Treatment

Once you have gathered all the data, you are ready to prepare a programme for treatment. You can use a form such as the one in figure 9.5 to create your programme. Following is an explanation of the various fields on the form.

- *Subjective:* This section documents how the client feels and what he or she reports to you before treatment; it also documents that the client consents to treatment.

- *Objective:* This section is about your observations as a therapist, including observations noted on the body map as well as data from the postural assessment, ROM, special tests and whatever you discover through palpation.

- *Treatment:* This section includes a list of what you did and how you did it.

- *Assessment:* This section describes your assessment of the treatment carried out. Here you note plans to retest if necessary to see if you have met your treatment goals.

- *Plan:* In this section, you can respond to questions such as *What do you intend to do for the next treatment session, and when is it to be?* and *Is there any aftercare advice you need to give your client?*

PROGRAMME FOR TREATMENT

Client Name:_____ Date:_____

Main problem:

Special notes:

Aims of treatment:

Subjective

Objective

Treatment

Assessment

Plan

Signature of client: _____

Figure 9.5 You can use a form such as this one to design a treatment programme for your client.

From J. Johnson, *Soft Tissue and Trigger Point Release,* 2nd ed. (Champaign, IL: Human Kinetics, 2019).

Case Studies

Following are assessments for four different clients, Client A, Client B, Client C and Client D. Look through them and then refer to their corresponding treatment plans. Can you see how the assessments helped influence the type of STR provided for each?

Client A

Client A presented with pain, stiffness and reduced ROM in the knee 2 weeks after being discharged from hospital following total knee replacement surgery. Client A's intake forms are shown in figures 9.6 to 9.9 at the end of the chapter.

CLIENT A'S INFORMATION

The following is a summary of Client A's intake forms:

- *Initial questions* (see figure 9.6): From these initial questions, vital information was gained that helped shape the treatment programme. For example, the problem clearly affected the client's daily activities. She had difficulty going down stairs and was unable to walk her dog. Nevertheless, she may not have wanted to do her physiotherapy exercises because they aggravated her pain. However, she is determined to get better; she is massaging her own knee and doing some of the mobilization exercises. It could be inferred that she wants some help increasing her knee flexibility, perhaps by doing something less painful than the exercises she has been prescribed. It is certain that she likes walking and is used to regular exercise with her dog, which may prove to be an important motivating factor. The fact that she has had this operation before on the other knee suggests she is familiar with the rehabilitation process for this particular condition, although she may be frustrated at not recovering as quickly as last time.

- *Medical history* (see figure 9.7): The main finding is that she has unmedicated high blood pressure. This finding is significant because after such surgery, there is often a period of recovery when the client is less active than usual and may gain weight. It often occurs with previously active clients, as in this case. Weight gain can increase blood pressure. It is therefore quite important that this client regain her mobility as soon as possible without too much exertion (exercise also increases blood pressure). Although the client has not reported feeling stressed, she shows a hint of anxiety concerning the fact that her previous recovery seemed to be quicker. Stress can also increase blood pressure, because tense muscles restrict capillary flow. The good news is that massage is believed to lower blood pressure, so it may be useful to use STR with massage.

Also significant is that the client had successful total knee replacement surgery to her left knee 2 years ago. This finding suggests that she is aware of the rehabilitation process and may understand the importance of carrying out the physiotherapy exercises (despite not liking them). Even though massage therapists don't usually prescribe exercises, a massage therapist can sometimes play an important role in encouraging clients to carry out the exercise programme that has been set by the physiotherapist or clinical exercise trainer. Knowing that the client has been receiving treatment from another practitioner (a physiotherapist), it is important to gain approval for massage and STR. In certain cases, stretching could be counterproductive to an existing treatment, so it is always best to get permission and advice if necessary before starting a treatment. As you know, it is also a professional courtesy.

Current medications include analgesics for knee pain. This finding is also important, for you need to know that a client can feel the depth of pressure of your locks, even when they are gentle, and any form of massage is contraindicated for clients who are taking painkillers of any kind. It also means that you need to warn the client that she should not take painkillers before treatment. It gives the client the opportunity to decline treatment should she feel the need to take painkillers. Nothing else was significant, and there were no contraindications to massage.

- *Body map* (see figure 9.8). The client has a longitudinal anterior scar on each knee. Using the map and medical history, it is easy to identify that the knee is the main problem area (though not necessarily the area to be treated), and that the scars represent surgical intervention. The right knee is visibly swollen. In addition to pain, this is likely to be a factor limiting flexibility.

- *Visual analogue scale* (see figure 9.8). The client's main problem is pain, and she has marked a point corresponding to level 7 on a pain scale of 0 to 10, where 10 is the worst pain. This pain score is quite high. It suggests careful management is needed, for although you do not know how irritable the knee is (that is, how quickly the pain comes on), you know that it is aggravated by weight bearing, so helping the client on and off the couch and not moving her about too much once she is on it may be important.

- *Postural assessment:* Client appears overweight. Scars show that the client has had knee operations; both knees have anterior longitudinal scars. Swelling to the right in anterior, posterior and lateral views indicates that the inflammatory process is active and that it may limit treatment.

- *Range of motion and other special tests:* Active and passive knee flexion were tested in sitting, supine and prone. All were uncomfortable, with flexion—both actively and passively—being the worst. The client preferred to have the ROM tests in prone despite having an anterior knee scar. This finding was interesting and useful because it indicated that STR to the hamstrings could be performed with the client in the prone position.

- *Palpation:* The client had slight soreness close to the scar but no other pain on palpation of the surrounding tissues.

CLIENT A'S PROGRAMME FOR TREATMENT
Figure 9.9 shows the treatment programme that was designed for Client A. The main aim was to help the client gain an increase in right knee flexion and extension. Notice that although STR to the quadriceps could have been used, this was inadvisable due to the recent surgery. Therefore, STR was only applied to the hamstring muscles, increasing extension of the knee joint. As part of the treatment, the therapist gently increased the point to which the knee was flexed, distracting

the client by gently shaking the limb. The overall effect was to gain 5 degrees flexion to the knee in prone and reduce feelings of discomfort at the back of the knee when the client was sitting with her legs outstretched, knees in extension.

The client was seen each day for 5 days initially, then once a week for 3 weeks. It is unusual for clients to come for treatment daily. However, this client was particularly keen to progress through her treatment quickly; because the treatment was light, not of long duration and resulted in an increased range of motion, albeit small, regular sessions seemed appropriate in this case. After five sessions, the client was advised to abstain from treatment, continue with self-massage and the physiotherapy exercises and apply cold to the knee if necessary.

Client B

Client B was a runner who came for treatment because his hamstrings and calves were feeling increasingly tight. Now that you have seen an example of different aspects of consultation, compare the Client A example with the information for this second client. The treatment programme (figure 9.10) and summaries of the findings from the initial questions, medical questionnaire and assessments have been provided. Can you see how all the assessments help determine not only whether you use STR at all, but which form of STR might be used and how frequently?

CLIENT B'S INFORMATION
The following is a summary of Client B's intake forms.

- *Initial questions:* This client had started running 4 weeks before and had experienced increasing tightness in his hamstrings and calves. The feeling of stiffness came on gradually, as might be expected, and was getting worse. It is aggravated by running and sitting for long periods, and although initially alleviated by hot baths, now seems to be constant. Importantly, the client does not report any pain. The client may have pulled his hamstring muscle in a football match 2 years ago but cannot remember exactly when this happened. He has tried some stretches he found in a book, but they gave him a backache. This seems like a straightforward case, with the treatment likely to be localized to the lower limbs. It may be worth taking a look at what sorts of stretches the client has been doing.

- *Medical history:* Client B experiences tension headaches (possibly related to his use of a computer for long hours), but there was nothing else significant and no contraindications to massage. Neck and shoulder tension can be treated with STR; this was noted for future reference but is not intended as part of this first treatment.

- *Body map:* The posterior of both lower limbs was shaded on this map, showing clearly where the main problem was. The fact that the client experiences tension headaches could have been noted on this map as a secondary problem.

- *Visual analogue scales:* Four VASs were used with this client to represent each of the lower limb muscles where he was experiencing stiffness (the hamstrings and calf on both the right and left leg). Interestingly, he reported a greater sensation of stiffness in the left hamstrings (5 on the scale), possibly where he had experienced a previous injury, and in the right calf (6 on the scale), perhaps because he is bearing more weight on his right side to compensate for the decreased functioning of the left hamstring. The VAS was 4 for the right hamstring and 4 for the left calf. It was noted, too, that the client's sensation of stiffness went all the way down to his Achilles tendon on both sides.

- *Postural assessment:* This assessment revealed that Client B stood slightly slumped, possibly with a mild degree of knee flexion on both sides. Assessment was difficult because the client reported feeling 'uncomfortable' standing in an upright posture; standing with straight legs seemed to aggravate tension in the hamstrings. Because the client reported that he was seated at work all day, an observation of his seated posture was carried out. This observation revealed that he liked to sit with his knees flexed, his ankles hooked onto the base of the chair in a position he reported as 'very comfortable'.

- *Range of motion and other special tests:* The straight-leg raise was used in testing the length of the client's hamstring muscles. Findings were 70 degrees on the left leg and 65 degrees on the right leg, with the client reporting an almost immediate increase in tension on both sides during the test. It was expected given that the client sits in knee flexion for about 6 hours a day at work. A differentiation test was carried out with the client standing to test the gastrocnemius and soleus muscles. There was decreased dorsiflexion on both sides and a shortened soleus on the right.

- *Palpation:* This assessment was done without oil. There was increased tension in the hamstrings and the calf muscles on both sides. There was a palpable mass of what may be scar tissue in the belly of the left biceps femoris muscle, which supports the client's report of a possible earlier injury.

CLIENT B'S PROGRAMME FOR TREATMENT

Based on the information provided, a programme for treatment was designed for Client B (see figure 9.10). The main aim of treatment was to decrease feelings of tension in the client's hamstring and calf muscles. Although a straight-leg raise test was used in assessing hamstring length, and it improved disproportionately after treatment of both sides, increasing hamstring length was not the main aim of the treatment. The VAS was used to help the client report his feelings of muscle stiffness. His main concern was not to have longer hamstrings but to feel less stiff; he was worried that stiffness might prevent him from continuing with his new running programme.

This case is a good example of how active STR might be applied effectively in addition to weekly massage. In this case, it was important to explain to the client the importance of avoiding active STR before running because active STR might decrease his muscle power. It was also important for him to be cautious about applying active STR too deeply immediately after a run, because there may be initially masked micro tears in the muscle that could be made worse with the deep pressure of the tennis ball. Active hamstring and calf stretches were applied as an alternative to post-exercise STR.

The client was then seen once per week for 4 weeks, and similar treatments were carried out. Feelings of stiffness decreased in both lower limbs. Post-exercise stretching was encouraged, and it was suggested that the client take advice on his seated posture at work. Although findings for the straight-leg raise did not alter much, there was a marked increase in ankle dorsiflexion, indicating increased flexibility in calf tissues.

The following two case studies, Client C and Client D, illustrate how STR might be used to help deactivate trigger points.

Client C

Client C presented with pain and reduced ROM in the upper trapezius and posterior shoulders.

CLIENT C'S INFORMATION
The following is a summary of Client C's intake forms.

- *Initial questions:* This client had been a call centre operative for over 3 years and was stationary at a desk, wearing a telephone headset. In the last 12 months he had begun to experience periods of neck and shoulder pain, which he was able to alleviate by moving the head and shoulders. However, the frequency and duration of pain episodes had increased and was getting worse. Pain was initially of a low level, described as 'uncomfortable', lasting only a few minutes and not coming on until the end of the day, alleviated by movement. At the time of the consultation pain was 'intense', came on within typing for 60 minutes and could not be alleviated with movement or stretching. The client had tried using a hot pack, which initially eased symptoms but now made little difference and he was worried he may have a serious neck and shoulder problem.

- *Medical history:* Client C had fusion of his L4/L5 vertebrae 10 years ago following a road traffic accident and used a rise–fall desk at work as prolonged sitting or prolonged standing of over 30 minutes caused low-back pain. There are no contraindications to upper-body massage.

- *Body map:* The client used the body map to shade in where he was feeling pain. Pain was noted to be in the upper part of trapezius radiating down the medial border of the scapula and into the back of the shoulder.

- *Visual analogue scales:* This client was unable to convert his pain sensation to a VAS, so it was not used.

- *Postural assessment:* This assessment revealed that Client C had a marked forward-head posture. An observation of both the standing and seated posture of this client was carried out. Standing posture revealed no issues, but it was observed that when seated at his work station the client's monitor was too high and the top of the monitor was not at the level of his eyes, causing the client to hold his head tilted back slightly.

- *Range of motion and other special tests:* Active neck ROM was carried out and revealed no restrictions in flexion or extension, although both were accompanied with 'bad' pain that felt 'muscular', whilst there was a limitation of at least 30 percent in both right and left lateral flexion. Right and left rotation range was normal but accompanied with 'pain and pulling'. Active shoulder range was full on both left and right sides, but elevation above 90 degrees caused pain in the upper trapezius on both sides with the client flexing his head as he attempted full elevation.

■   *Palpation:* Palpation revealed an active trigger point in levator scapulae, which reproduced the client's pain on both left and right sides. He had some tenderness at the base of the skull.

CLIENT C'S PROGRAMME FOR TREATMENT
Based on the information provided, a programme for treatment was designed for Client C (figure 9.11). Aims of the treatment were to *(1)* increase the time by which pain came on at work from 60 minutes to anything above this time, *(2)* reduce the severity of pain, *(3)* reduce the length of time the client experienced pain during a pain episode, *(4)* reduce the frequency of pain episodes and *(5)* improve lateral ROM in the neck and for rotation to be less painful with less of a pulling sensation.

Client D

Client D presented with pain in the left arm radiating into the left thumb and forefinger.

CLIENT D'S INFORMATION
The following is a summary of Client D's intake forms.

■   *Initial questions:* This client was a bariatric client who was housebound. She was unemployed, awaiting surgery as part of a weight management programme and under the supervision of a local doctor who was present at the time of the initial consultation; the doctor had ruled out angina or heart issues as being the cause of the left arm pain, believing it to be muscular in origin. The doctor recommended massage as a possible solution. Left arm pain was preventing the client from doing crochet, a hobby about which she was passionate.

■   *Medical history:* Client D reported her weight to be '27 stones' (171 kilos; 377 lb) and they were taking aspirin daily. She also took thyroxine daily for hypothyroidism.

■   *Body map:* The client used an enlarged image of the upper limb from a body map to shade in where she was feeling pain. Pain was noted to be in the front and back of the arm primarily, sometimes with sensations in the forearm, very occasionally right-sided chest pain. This client was noted as left-handed.

■   *Visual analogue scales:* This client reported pain as 'constant burning' and around 6 out of 10 on the VAS but rising to 8 to 9 when crocheting.

■   *Postural assessment:* This client was assessed when resting in her usual chair at home, a purpose built recliner. The chair was reclined to around 45 degrees from vertical, causing the client to adopt a position of marked neck flexion.

- *Range of motion and other special tests:* Range of motion in the neck and shoulder were not possible as the client was unable to sit upright. Active and passive ranges were performed for the elbow, wrist and finger of both hands. Supination was reduced and 'sore' in the left wrist; wrist and finger extension in the left wrist was full but described as 'tight' as was left thumb extension.

- *Palpation:* Palpation of the upper limb revealed mild tenderness throughout the anterior surface. It was not possible to palpate the posterior surface. Palpation did not reproduce the client's symptoms. However, palpation of the left scalenes did.

CLIENT D'S PROGRAMME FOR TREATMENT

Based on the information provided, a programme for treatment was designed for Client D (figure 9.12). Aims of the treatment were to reduce the frequency and intensity of pain in the left upper limb from 6 to 9 out of 10 on the VAS to below this number.

Closing Remarks

You should now have a good understanding of the importance of asking initial questions, and you have learned how a variety of different assessments can be used to help inform your treatments. The case studies illustrate different situations in which STR could help. Can you think of any of your own clients for whom STR might be appropriate? This chapter has given you some insight into the variety of assessments you could use with your clients; you are encouraged to try some of them.

Quick Questions

1. When asking your initial questions, what could you say instead of 'Where's the pain?'
2. If a client presents with more than one part of his or her body needing treatment, how might you quickly indicate in your records which area is the main area of treatment?
3. What does VAS stand for?
4. In the programme for treatment, what does the subjective information tell you?
5. In the programme for treatment, what does the objective information tell you?

INITIAL QUESTIONS

1. How may I help?

Looking for pain relief. Hoping massage therapy will help.

2. Where is the discomfort you described?

Pain in right knee.

3. When did it start?

Following recent total knee replacement surgery to that side.

4. How was it caused?

As above.

5. Is it getting better, worse or staying the same?

Better—slowly.

6. Does anything make it worse?

Doing the physiotherapy exercises to encourage flexion/extension!

7. Does anything make it better?

Not doing the physiotherapy exercises! For self-management, the client uses painkillers; self-massage to whole of knee avoiding anterior wound; mobilization within pain-free range.

8. Have you had previous treatment for this complaint? Was it helpful?

No. However, left knee replaced 2 years ago and seemed to recover more quickly.

9. Have you had this condition before?

n/a

10. Have you had any previous injuries to the same area?

Severe osteoarthritis, hence total knee replacement operation.

11. Can you describe the type of discomfort you are feeling?

Pain (level 7 VAS) on active and passive movement of knee, especially flexion; stiffness.

12. How does this condition affect your work and leisure?

Unable to walk dog; difficulty in all daily activities involving walking and stairs.

13. Is there anything else you think I need to know?

Client reports pain as 'burning' when attempting physical therapy exercises; this changes to 'aching' after exercise and may last several hours.

Figure 9.6 Client A's initial responses to questions.

MEDICAL HISTORY

Name: Client A	Tel. No. (home) :	Tel. No. (work):
Address:	Mobile No.:	Date of birth: May 1936

Dr's name/tel no:

Address:

Occupation: retired school cook	Weight: 70 kg Height: 5 ft 6 in. (168 cm)
Current medication: analgesics for postop pain	Referred? No
Recent operations/illnesses: total right knee replacement	Pregnancy:
Circulation problems: (heart, pulmonary oedema, high/low blood pressure, poor circulation)	Unmedicated high blood pressure
Respiratory system: (asthma, bronchitis, hayfever)	None
Skin disorders: (dermatitis, eczema, sensitivity, fungal infections)	None
Muscular or skeletal problems: (fibromyalgia, previous fractures)	Stiffness and swelling in right knee following recent operation, with decreased range of motion
Neurological problems: (sciatica, epilepsy, migraine)	None
Urinary problems: (cystitis, thrush, kidney problems)	None
Immune system: (prone to colds, reduced immune status)	None
Gynaecological problems: (PMT, menopause, HRT, irregular periods)	None
Hormonal problems: (diabetes)	None
Digestive problems: (indigestion, constipation, IBS)	None
Stress-related or psychological problems: (depression, anxiety, panic attacks, mood swings)	None

INDEMNITY: I confirm to the best of my knowledge that I have not withheld any information relevant to my treatment and that I understand and accept full responsibility for the treatment that I am given. I also agree that I have given the correct information as detailed on this form, and shall inform the therapist should these circumstances change.

Client signature:_____

Therapist signature _____ Date _____

Figure 9.7 Client A's medical history.

ASSESSMENTS FOR CLIENT A

Visual Analogue Scale

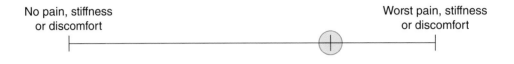

No pain, stiffness
or discomfort

Worst pain, stiffness
or discomfort

Body Map

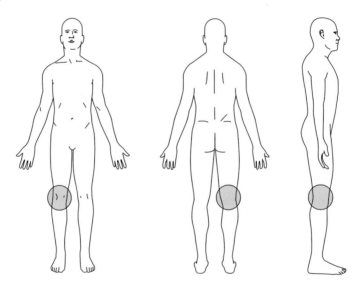

Figure 9.8 Client A's VAS and body map.

PROGRAMME FOR TREATMENT

Client Name: Client A   Date: /   /

Main problem: Pain and stiffness in right knee following total knee replacement surgery.
Special notes: Consent for treatment given by physiotherapist; pain worsened following
   physiotherapy treatment to encourage ROM at knee.
Aims of treatment: Assist client in achieving flexion/extension at the knee as recommended by physiotherapist, beginning with flexion.

Subjective

Client well and consents to treatment plan. No pain in knee at present.
VAS for previous pain (see consultation).

Objective

Swollen right knee.
Longitudinal anterior scars both knees.
Limited active and passive flexion and extension when tested in sitting, supine and
   prone positions, with localized pain reported most on flexion.
Client has difficulty getting onto and off treatment couch. In prone, knee flexion limited
   (by pain) to 80 degrees.

Treatment

Gentle passive flexion and extension of knee joint in prone.
Passive STR through clothing to left hamstrings in prone to demonstrate technique.
   Approx 2 min.
Passive soft tissue release to right hamstrings in prone. Approx 4 min (initially was
   uncomfortable to anterior knee, so continued with bolster beneath knee, just superior
   to scar).
Technique repeated for 4 more min whilst gently shaking client's leg during knee exten-
   sion. Each time, the knee was flexed passively a degree more.
Client advised to rest with legs raised to encourage lymphatic drainage to aid reduction
   in swelling.

Assessment

Demonstrating on client's left leg helped me gain her confidence.
Using a bolster to prevent the knee from touching the treatment couch worked well.
   Client much enjoyed the gentle shaking of the leg during the application.
Knee flexion increased by 5 degrees due to passive flexion.
Client reported being 'amazed' at her increase in flexion. In supine, resting knee exten-
   sion was reported as 'more comfortable'.

Plan

10 min STR daily as previously noted. Client to rest in position shown. Client to continue with daily physiotherapy exercises.
Attempt muscle energy technique to quadriceps whilst sitting as adjunct to STR.

Signature of client: _____

Figure 9.9   Client A's programme for treatment, which incorporates subjective and objective
information as well as information related to treatment, assessment and the plan.

PROGRAMME FOR TREATMENT

Client Name: Client B   Date: /   /

Main problem: Tight calves and hamstrings.
Special notes: Client wants to continue with running programme 4 times per week.
  Aims of treatment: Decrease feelings of stiffness in hamstrings and calves.

Subjective

Client well and consents to treatment plan.

Objective

Decreased passive straight-leg raise (SLR) both sides (70 degrees L, 65 degrees R).
  Decreased ankle dorsiflexion both sides.
VAS for stiffness (see consultation).
Small, palpable, nonpainful mass left biceps femoris.

Treatment

Basic warm-up massage to posterior of both lower limbs prior to treatment with STR
  approx 5 min each side.
In prone, feet off couch, 5 min active-assisted STR to hamstrings and 5 min active-
  assisted STR to calf on each side through towel. Further, deeper massage to posterior
  lower limb (2 min) then STR repeated through towel 3 min hamstrings, 3 min calf each
  side. Massage again 2 min each side.
In supine, massage to quads and tibialis anterior both sides, approx 10 min each side.
Active STR for hamstrings and calves demonstrated to client and client given hard
  tennis ball to use for this purpose. Caution regarding pre- and post-exercise use of STR
  explained.
Active post-exercise hamstring and calf stretches demonstrated to client.

Assessment

SLR following treatment = 75 degrees L, 75 degrees R. Increased dorsiflexion when
  tested actively.
Client perceives less tension both legs.
Overall initial treatment appears effective in decreasing client's feelings of stiffness in
  hamstrings and calves.

Plan

Massage as noted once per week.
Client to practise active STR and stretches as advised.
Client to consider treatment to whole of lower limb both sides as maintenance/prophy-
  lactic massage whilst on running programme.

Signature of client: _____

Figure 9.10 Client B's programme for treatment, which incorporates subjective and
objective information as well as information related to treatment, assessment and the plan.

PROGRAMME FOR TREATMENT

Client Name: Client C   Date: /   /

Main problem: neck and bilateral posterior shoulder pain.
Special notes: Client unable to sit for more than 30 minutes without low-back pain.

Subjective

Client well and consents to treatment plan.

Objective

Decreased active cervical lateral flexion by 30 percent both L and R sides.
Active cervical rotation full L and R but painful with pulling.
Active cervical flexion and extension full with pain on extension.
Active triggers found in levator scapulae L and R.
Active shoulder range full with upper trapezius pain above 90 degrees abduction bilaterally.

Treatment

Client seated on inclined massage chair in therapy room at work. Basic warm-up massage to posterior of both shoulders and neck for approx 5 min each side.
STR to deactivate trigger points treated on both left and right levator scapulae interspersed with effleurage and light pettrisage massage for a total of 20 minutes.
In standing, client taught active neck stretches for levator scapulae.
Client advised re positioning of monitor when standing at work station. Advice given regards levator scapulae stretching.

Assessment

Active cervical ROM: Minor improvement in lateral and rotation ranges but client reports much reduced sensation of pain and pulling. Active shoulder ROM uncomfortable past 90 degrees of abduction but no longer painful.
Overall initial treatment appears effective in decreasing client's feelings of pain and pulling neck muscles, and pain in posterior shoulder.

Plan

Treatment as noted twice per week at work.
Client to practise levator scapulae stretches as advised.
Client to adjust standing work station posture. (Check this next appointment).
Client to be taught neck retraction exercises.

Signature of client: _____

Figure 9.11   Client C's programme for treatment, which incorporates subjective and objective information as well as information related to treatment, assessment and the plan.

PROGRAMME FOR TREATMENT

Client Name: Client D   Date: /   /

Main problem: pain in the left upper limb.

Special notes: Client is bariatric, unable to sit upright and needs to be treated in chair in client's home.

Subjective

Client's doctor confirms left-sided pain is of muscular origin. Client consents to treatment plan.

Objective

Active and passive elbow, wrist and finger of both hands. Supination mildly reduced and 'sore' in the left wrist; wrist and finger extension in the left wrist full but 'tight' as is left thumb extension.

Treatment

Client seated at home in specialized chair. Incline of the chair was altered to enable client to sit more upright and facilitate treatment to scalenes but note full upright position is not possible for this client. STR to deactivate trigger points in left scalenes was attempted but unsuccessful as this made client feel nauseous. Active STR trigger points in scalenes was taught to client. Client advised to maintain more upright position where possible and explanations given with regards head posture and referred pain from scalenes. Active stretches for the wrist and finger flexors was taught. 10 minutes effleurage to anterior of left arm and anterior and posterior of left forearm followed by a total of 10 minutes of passive stretches of wrist pronators and wrist and finger flexors. Diary given to client to record active trigger point release to scalenes and symptoms. Reduced intensity of crocheting advised, interspersed with other sedentary activities.

Assessment

Only minor improvement in symptoms, but client education went well. Client understood how to identify trigger points in scalenes and agreed to work these during the week.

Plan

Revisit client once per week to monitor effect of active STR to scalenes and active wrist and finger stretches.

Client to practise deactivation of trigger points in scalenes as advised.

Client to practise wrist and finger stretches as advised.

Signature of client: _____

Figure 9.12   Client D's programme for treatment, which incorporates subjective and objective information as well as information related to treatment, assessment and the plan.

Answers to Quick Questions

Chapter 1

1. STR targets specific areas of tension within a muscle, whereas general stretching works on the whole muscle.
2. You can lock a muscle using a forearm, fist, elbow or massage tool.
3. When applying a lock, start at the proximal end.
4. STR should be used cautiously in a pre-event setting because stretching temporarily decreases muscle power.
5. STR may be applied post-event but should not be too deep because there may be microtrauma, the sensation of which may be masked by an increased level of natural endorphins.
6. Muscular problems associated with trigger points:
   - Tight and weak muscles
   - Decreased muscular strength
   - Muscle pain
7. Joint problems associated with trigger points
   - Stiff joints
   - Joint pain

Chapter 2

1. You could use your palm to lock tissues when you need a gentle lock, such as when applying STR as a pre- or post-event treatment.
2. STR is not appropriate for the following kinds of clients:
   - Someone for whom general massage is contraindicated
   - Someone who bruises easily
   - Someone with hypermobility syndrome
3. The three types of STR are passive, active-assisted and active.
4. You do not hold a lock at the end of a stretch; once the tissues have stretched, you remove your lock.
5. To measure the effectiveness of STR you could
   - ask for feedback from the client regarding pain sensation before and after treatment;
   - use a visual analogue scale; and
   - do movement tests, such as the straight leg raise or prone knee bend.

Chapter 3

1. When a muscle is in a neutral position, the fibres are neither shortened too much nor stretched.
2. The therapist performs the stretch in passive STR.
3. Yes, a lock is maintained whilst a muscle is being stretched.
4. Clients are most likely to feel the stretch as you approach the distal end of the muscle.
5. You need to be careful when applying passive STR with oil massage because working through a towel onto skin that has been oiled provides an extremely firm lock.

Chapter 4

1. Both the client and the therapist work together to achieve active-assisted STR: The therapist provides the lock whilst the client moves to produce the stretch.
2. Active-assisted STR is useful for treating clients who find it difficult to relax during treatment and for those who like to be engaged with their treatment.
3. Active-assisted STR is a useful form of rehabilitation after joint immobilization because it increases joint range and helps strengthen surrounding muscles.
4. The biggest difference between passive and active-assisted STR is that in passive STR, the relaxed muscles are being stretched; in active-assisted STR, the muscle being stretched is often contracting eccentrically.
5. Some clients get confused if the therapist swaps between passive and active-assisted STR because one requires them to move and one does not.

Chapter 5

1. You concentrically contract the muscle you want to work on in order to shorten it.
2. You contract the muscle first, then lock the soft tissues.
3. You place your first lock nearest to the origin of the muscle and work towards the distal end.
4. It is best to avoid STR if you bruise easily. Because it is necessary to apply fairly strong locks, these could induce unintentional bruising.
5. When you are first learning the technique, apply STR for only two to three minutes on the same area.

Chapter 6

1. In passive STR to the rhomboids, the scapula needs to protract in order to bring about the stretch. The arm, therefore, needs to be positioned off the couch at the start of the treatment.
2. To dissipate the pressure of any lock, work through a folded towel or facecloth.
3. Active-assisted STR is a safe method of stretching tissues of the neck because the stretch is performed by the client himself or herself, and it is likely the client will stretch only within his or her pain-free range.
4. Be aware of the clavicle and acromion process and avoid pressing into these when applying active-assisted STR to the upper fibres of the trapezius.
5. Once you have locked the tissues to the erector spinae with the client in extension, the client flexes forward, thus bringing about a stretch.

Chapter 7

1. When treating hamstrings passively, avoid locking into the popliteal space behind the knee.
2. Ankle plantar flexors are very strong muscles, so it requires more force to dorsiflex the ankle passively and stretch those muscles. Using your thigh provides greater force and is safer for you than using your hand.
3. Never stand on a ball when performing active STR because doing so could be dangerous. Always apply the technique sitting down.
4. Clients with flat feet (that is, those whose ankles are everted) often feel STR to the peroneals more acutely than do other clients.
5. STR to the iliacus is applied with the client in side lying.

Chapter 8

1. STR to the triceps is felt particularly after activities that involve elbow extension, such as tennis, doing shoulder presses and polishing.
2. Passive STR to the triceps is performed with the client in prone and with his or her forearm off the couch.
3. When performing active STR to wrist extensors, start with your wrist in extension.
4. When performing active-assisted STR to wrist flexors, you lock in near the elbow.
5. Activities such as typing, driving and golf require wrist and finger flexion, and anyone who performs these activities is likely to benefit from STR to the wrist flexors.

Chapter 9

1. As an alternative to *Where's the pain?* you might ask *How does that feel?*
2. When a client presents with more than one part of the body needing treatment, one way to quickly indicate which area is the main area for treatment is to use a body map and mark the areas as (1), (2), (3) and so on, with (1) as the most important or main area.
3. VAS stands for visual analogue scale.
4. In the programme for treatment, the subjective information tells you what the client has said and how the client feels.
5. In the programme for treatment, the objective information records your observations as a therapist and includes information from the body map, postural assessment, ROM testing, special tests and whatever you discover on palpation.

References

Chapter 1

American College of Sports Medicine. (2018). ACSM issues new recommendations on quality and quantity of exercise. Retrieved from www.acsm.org/about-acsm/media-room/news-releases/2011/08/01/acsm-issues-new-recommendations-on-quantity-and-quality-of-exercise

Chaitow, L. (2000). *Modern neuromuscular techniques*. London, England: Churchill Livingstone.

Davies, C. (2004). *The trigger point therapy workbook* (2nd ed.). Oakland, CA: New Harbinger.

Simons, D.G., Travell, J.G., & Simons, L.S. (1999). *Travell and Simons' myofascial pain and dysfunction: The trigger point manual. Vol 1: Upper half of body* (2nd ed.). Baltimore, MD: Lippincott Williams & Wilkins.

Stanton, T., Moseley, G., Wong, A., & Gregory, N. (2017). Feeling stiffness in the back: A protective perceptual inference in chronic pain. *Scientific Reports, 7*(1): 9681. Retrieved from www.nature.com/articles/s41598-017-09429-1

Chapter 6

Botha, D. (2017). A comparison between ischemic compression and foam rolling in the treatment of active rhomboid trigger points. University of Johannesburg. Abstract retrieved from https://ujcontent.uj.ac.za/vital/access/manager/Repository/uj:25556

Cummings, M. (2003). Myofascial pain from pectoralis major following trans-axillary surgery. *Acupuncture in Medicine, 21*(3): 105-107. Retrieved from http://aim.bmj.com/content/21/3/105

De Meulemeester, K., Castelein, B., Coppieters, I., Barbe, T., Cools, A., & Cagnie, B. (2017). Comparing trigger point dry needling and manual pressure technique for the management of myofascial neck/shoulder pain: A randomized clinical trial. *Journal of Manipulative and Physical Therapeutics, 40*(1): 11-20.

Fernandes-de-las-Peñas, C., Layton, M., & Dommerholt, J. (2015). Dry needling for the management of thoracic spine pain. *Journal of Manual Manipulative Therapy, 23*(3): 147-153. Retrieved from www.tandfonline.com/doi/abs/10.1179/2042618615Y.0000000001?journalCode=yjmt20

Florencio, L., Giantomassi, M., Carvalho, G., Goncalves, M., Dach, F., Fernandez-de-las-Penas, C., & Bevilaqua-Grossi, D. (2015). Generalized pressure pain hypersensitivity in the cervical muscles in women with migraine. *Pain Medicine, 16*: 1629-1634.

Johnson, J. (2012). *Postural assessment*. Champaign, IL: Human Kinetics.

Lee, J., Hwang, S., Han, S., & Han, D. (2016). Effects of stretching the scalene muscles on slow vital capacity. *Journal of Physical Therapy Science, 28*: 1825-1828. doi:10.1589/jpts.28.1825

Moraska, A., Schmiege, S., Mann, J., Butryn, N., & Krutsch, J. (2017). Responsiveness of myofascial trigger points to single and multiple trigger point release massages. *American Journal of Physical Medicine and Rehabilitation, 96*: 639-645. Retrieved from www.ajpmr.com

Robbins, M.S., Kuruvilla, D., Blumenfeld, A., Charleston, I.V., Sorrell, M., Robertson, C.E., . . . Ashkenazi, A. (2014). Trigger point injections for headache disorders: Expert consensus methodology and narrative review. *The Journal of Head and Face Pain, 54*(9): 1441-1459. doi:10.1111/head.12442

Shin, J.K., Shin, J.C., Kim, W.S., Chang, W.H., & Lee, S.H. (2014). Application of ultrasound-guided trigger point injection for myofascial trigger points in the subscapularis and pectoralis muscles to post-mastectomy patients: A pilot study. *Yonsei Medical Journal, 55*(3): 792-799. doi:10.3349/ymj.2014.55.3.792

Simons, D.G., Travell, J.G., & Simons, L.S. (1999). *Travell and Simons' myofascial pain and dysfunction: The trigger point manual. Vol 1: Upper half of body* (2nd ed.). Baltimore, MD: Lippincott Williams & Wilkins.

Taleb, W., Youssef, A., & Saleh, A. (2016). The effectiveness of manual versus algometer pressure release techniques for treating active myofascial trigger points of the upper trapezius. *Journal of Bodywork and Movement Therapies, 20*: 863-869.

Tewari, S., Madabushi, M., Agarwal, A., Gautam, S., & Khuba S. (2017). Chronic pain in a patient with Ehlers-Danlos syndrome (hypermobility type): The role of myofascial trigger point injections. *Journal of Bodywork and Movement Therapies, 21*: 194-196.

Chapter 7

Espí-López, G., Serra-Año, P., Vicent-Ferrando, J., Sanchez-Moreno-Giner, M., Arias-Buria, J., Cleland, J., & Fernández-de-las-Peñas, C. (2017). Effectiveness of inclusion of dry needling in a multimodal therapy program for patellofemoral pain: A randomized parallel-group trial. *Journal of Orthopaedic and Sport and Physical Therapy, 47*(6): 392-401.

Ferguson, L. (2014). Adult idiopathic scoliosis: The tethered spine. *Journal of Bodywork and Movement Therapies, 18*: 99-111.

Grieve, R., Barnett, S., Coghill, N., & Cramp, F. (2013). Myofascial trigger point therapy for triceps surae dysfunction: A case series. *Manual Therapy, 18*(6): 519-525.

Grieve, R., Cranston, A., Henderson, A., John, R., Malone, G., & Mayall, C. (2013). The immediate effect of triceps surae myofascial trigger point therapy on restricted active ankle joint dorsiflexion in recreational runners: A crossover randomised controlled trial. *Journal of Bodywork and Movement Therapies, 17*: 453-461.

Huguenin, L., Brukner, P., McCrory, P., Smith, P., Wajswelner, H., & Bennell, K. (2005). Effect of dry needling of gluteal muscles on straight leg raise: A randomised, placebo controlled, double blind trial. *British Journal of Sports Medicine, 39*: 84-90.

Oh, S., Kim, M., Lee, M., Lee, D., Kim, T., & Yoon B. (2016). Self-management of myofascial trigger point release by using an inflatable ball among elderly patients with chronic low back pain: A case series. *Annals of Yoga and Physical Therapy, 1*(3): 1013.

Patel, D., Vyas, N., & Sheth, M. (2016). Immediate effect of application of bilateral self myofascial release on the plantar surface of the foot on hamstring and lumbar spine flexibility: A quasi experimental study. *International Journal of Therapeutic Applications, 32*: 94-99.

Pavkovich, R. (2015). The use of dry needling for a subject with chronic lateral hip and thigh pain: A case report. *International Journal of Sports Physical Therapy, 10*(2): 246-255.

Renan-Ordine, R., Alburquerque-Sendin, F., de Souza, D., Cleland, J., & Fernandes-de-las-Peñas, C. (2011). Effectiveness of myofascial trigger point manual therapy combined with a self-stretching protocol for the management of plantar heel pain: A randomized controlled trial. *Journal of Orthopaedic and Sports Physical Therapy, 41*(2): 43-50.

Rossi, A., Blaustein, S., Brown, J., Dieffenderfer, K., Ervine, E., Griffin, S., Firierson, E., Geist, K., & Johanson, M. (2017). Spinal peripheral dry needling versus peripheral dry needling alone among individuals with a history of ankle sprain: A randomized controlled trial. *International Journal of Sports Physical Therapy, 12*(7): 1034-1047.

Trampas, A., Kitsios, A., Sykaras, E., Symeonidis, S., & Lararous, L. (2010). Clinical massage and modified proprioceptive neuromuscular facilitation stretching in males with latent myofascial trigger points. *Physical Therapy in Sport, 11*(3): 91-98.

Chapter 8

González-Iglesias, J., Cleland, J.A., del Rosario Gutierrez-Vega, M., & Fernández-de-las-Peñas, C. (2011). Multimodal management of lateral epicondylalgia in rock climbers: A prospective case series. *Journal of Manipulative and Physiological Therapeutics, 34*(9): 635-642.

Hidalgo-Lozano, A., Fernández-de-las-Peñas, C., Alonso-Blanco, C., Ge, H.-Y., Arendt-Nielsen, L., & Arroyo-Morales, L. (2010). Muscle trigger points and pressure pain hyperalgesia in the shoulder muscles in patients with unilateral shoulder impingement: A blinded, controlled study. *Experimental Brain Research, 202*: 915-925.

Nielsen, A. (1981). Case study: Myofascial pain of the posterior shoulder relieved by spray and stretch. *Journal of Orthopaedic and Sports Physical Therapy, 3*(1): 21-26.

Simons, D.G., Travell J.G., & Simons L.S. (1999). *Travell and Simons' myofascial pain and dysfunction: The trigger point manual. Vol 1: Upper half of body* (2nd ed.). Baltimore, MD: Lippincott Williams & Wilkins.

Chapter 9

Gift, A. (1989). Visual analogue scales: Measurement of subjective phenomena. *Nursing Research, 38*(5): 286-287.

Hawker, G., Mian, S., Kendzerska, T., & French, M. (2011). Measures of adult pain. *Arthritis Care and Research, 63*(Suppl 11): S240-S252.

Johnson, J. (2012). *Postural assessment*. Champaign, IL: Human Kinetics.

Kahn, M. (2008). Etiquette-based medicine. *The New England Journal of Medicine, 358*(19): 1988-1989.

Kendall, F.P., McCreary, E.K., Provance, P.G., Rodgers, M.M., & Romani, W.A. (2005). *Muscles: Testing and function with posture and pain* (5th ed.). Baltimore, MD: Lippincott Williams & Wilkins.

Melzack, R. (1975). The McGill Pain Questionnaire: Major properties and scoring methods. *Pain, 1*(3): 277-299.

Rosenzveig, A., Kuspinar, A., Daskalopoulou, S., & Mayo, N. (2014). Toward patient-centered care: A systematic review of how to ask questions that matter to patients. *Medicine, 93*(22): 1-10.

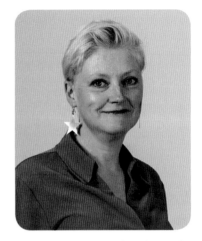

Jane Johnson, MSc, is a chartered physiotherapist and sport massage therapist specializing in musculoskeletal occupational health. She has been using and teaching soft tissue release (STR) for many years and has a thorough grounding in anatomy, which she uses to explain STR in straightforward terms. She has worked with numerous client groups, including athletes, recreational exercisers, office workers, and older adults; this experience has enabled her to adapt STR for various types of clients and provide practical tips for readers.

Johnson has taught continuing professional development workshops for many organizations in the United Kingdom and in other countries. This experience has brought her into contact with thousands of therapists of all disciplines and informed her own practice. She is passionate about supporting and inspiring newly qualified or less confident therapists so they feel more self-assured in their work. She frequently presents STR at conferences and exhibitions for therapists.

Johnson is a member of the Chartered Society of Physiotherapy and is registered with the Health and Care Professions Council. A member of the Medico Legal Association of Chartered Physiotherapists, she provides expert witness reports on cases involving soft tissue therapies.